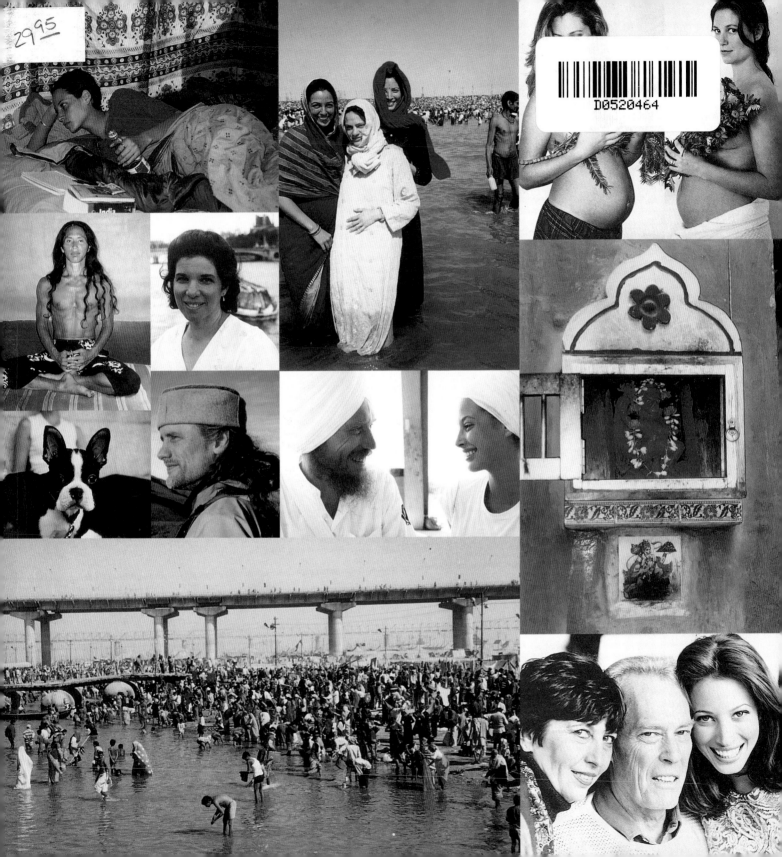

29.95

D0520464

LIVING YOGA

Creating a Life Practice

CHRISTY TURLINGTON

HYPERION

NEW YORK

Printed and bound in Great Britain by Butler & Tanner Limited,
Frome and London.

ISBN: 0-7868-6806-6

Hyperion books are available for special promotions and premiums.
For details contact Hyperion Special Markets, 77 W. 66th Street,
New York, New York 10023, or call 212-456-0100.

FIRST EDITION

Book design by Richard Oriolo

10   9   8   7   6   5   4   3   2   1

This book is dedicated to all my past, present, and future teachers,

as well as the teacher within whom I have too often ignored.

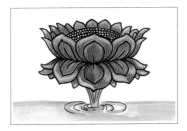

For those who so generously contributed to this book, especially Lisa Jacobson for pushing me to undertake this enormous project, to Sabrina Dupré for keeping me focused and supporting me along the way, and to E. B. for taking the knocks that came from the fears of swimming in foreign waters.

CONTENTS

PERSONAL JOURNEYS

FOREWORD

Living Yoga is a powerful inspiration for those of us who want to have their cake and eat it too. The cake here is a life of fulfillment, spiritual, yes, but not opposed to fulfillment on the human level. Eating it too is living in a way that material realities are mastered and turned into assets in a spiritual life that brings happiness to self and others.

Living Yoga shows us that the human being is both spiritual and material: You cannot neglect either dimension and expect the other one to flourish. If you are too spiritual—defined as someone who aims at another world, ignoring other persons and things in this world, not even caring for body or health—then you may have some far-out moments, but in the long run your life will be painful and isolated. If you are too material, you may win wealth, fame, and a superficial level of stressed-out energy; but you will get no satisfaction, you will inevitably reach a point where it will all seem vain and hollow, your relations with others will be shallow and unhappy, and ultimately you will find out that with worldly success or possession, you just "can't take it with you."

In *Living Yoga*, Christy shares with us her own journey and its striving for the union of the spiritual and the material in a life of true fulfillment on every level.

Too long have we been conditioned to consider that material and social fulfillment can only be achieved at the cost of spiritual development, that the two are drastically opposed —"Render the one unto Caesar . . . and the other to the Lord!" So we tend to live as if we were being chased by Caesar, or trying to become a Caesar, and we keep our dues to "the Lord" uneasily in the back of our minds until things go very wrong, we are deeply ill, a loved one has a catastrophe, or we are near death. Subliminally we have the image of Jesus rendering unto the Lord his body and his very life's breath, and we naturally shy away from such extreme sacrifice.

Christy's story is honest and moving, as is her explanation of the essence of the great Indian teaching of yoga: as "yoking," "joining," "uniting" life and spirituality, realizing the true aim of life of loving others wisely and being loved well in return, of sharing that love as creativity with the whole society, not out of greed for success but just naturally, for the sheer joy of it, and on top of that receiving the appreciation of others, good reputation, and even the financial rewards due to one who creates what people need and enjoy.

Not that Christy's journey is over, far from it; she is totally straightforward and honest about how much she has yet to experience and learn, and how much she wants to share and do for others in this world of struggle and inconceivable opportunity. She speaks to us not only from the mountaintop, but also from the streets filled with the dust of the collapsing towers of New York and the young girls' schoolyard in traumatized Afghanistan, not only from her personal success and fame, but also from her personal tragedies and anguish. Her instructions in the yogas that she has found useful speak to us out of her very humanness, making us feel that we too can take responsibility for our lives and turn body and mind realistically toward fulfillment.

There is the yoga of "Sun and Moon" (*Hatha*), the systematic spiritual and physical positioning of body and mind that comes from the sages of ancient India to help us harmonize our bodies with the environment and open our minds to our unlimited inner horizon of spiritual potential. There is Action (*Karma*) yoga, where our deeds in the world are dedicated to God or Buddha, the security of divine wisdom and the creativity of universal love for all beings. There is Wisdom (*Jnana*) yoga, where we are empowered to know from the depths of our being our real nature and our deep interconnectedness with all living beings, in order to feel the joy of "inter-being" with everything, nevermore to feel lost or lonely. There is Royal (*Raja*) yoga, the union of all our faculties and powers to realize our true destiny and bring help and happiness to others.

Living Yoga opens the door for us to all of these arts of living well and better, our heritage from the ancient sages brought to life and made relevant to us today through the inspiring example of Christy's own adventure. It is an honor and a pleasure to introduce it to you.

Robert A. F. Thurman
Jey Tsong Khapa Professor of
Indo-Tibetan Buddhist Studies
Columbia University;
President, Tibet House U.S.
April 22, 2002

The Journey

One day you finally knew
what you had to do, and began,
though the voices around you
kept shouting
their bad advice—
though the whole house
began to tremble
and you felt the old tug
at your ankles.
"Mend my life!"
each voice cried.
But you didn't stop.
You knew what you had to do,
though the wind pried
with its stiff fingers
at the very foundations,
though their melancholy
was terrible.
It was already late
enough, and a wild night,
and the road full of fallen
branches and stones.
But little by little,
as you left their voices behind,
the stars began to burn
through the sheets of clouds,
and there was a new voice
which you slowly
recognized as your own,
that kept you company
as you strode deeper and deeper
into the world,
determined to do
the only thing you could do—
determined to save
the only life you could save.

—MARY OLIVER

INTRODUCTION

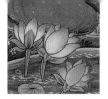

Eastern Philosophy says that human beings have forgotten what they came here for. With all the stimulation outside of ourselves, we have lost sight of the Beloved, our creator, and have lost ourselves as a result.

I truly believe that we have the answers within us, but it takes incredible discipline and hard work to gain back those abandoned gifts we were given as a birthright. Many of us have lost the ability to feel things, and look to others for clarification and purpose when the answers are deep inside of ourselves. We are each a part of our divine maker and creation itself, and when we accept that divine connection, we have begun upon the path of enlightenment.

Yoga allows us to experience this connection. Through the yoking of our bodies, minds, and hearts to a higher power of existence, we awaken the *shakti,* or spiritual energy hidden within, and our highest capabilities are revealed. With this realization comes a confidence, which cannot be destroyed. This is Self-realization. Once that connection is established, the source is accessible at any time to find the answers that we may be searching for. Through practicing yoga, you will also become more conscious of your behavior in the world, and how the behavior of things outside of yourself can affect you. You learn that you can go out into the world and affect others in a number of positive ways.

We are each born with unlimited potential and a deep inner knowledge of what is right and what is true, but life would be without meaning if we did not have to work (at least) a little toward this self-discovery. We are our own God-given tools to attain this knowledge and the freedom that will come when it is realized fully, so we must strengthen and sharpen our tools, in preparation for this divine union. This can only be achieved through practice, and yoga is essentially the practice of refining ourselves holistically and specifically for this deeply spiritual purpose. Yoga is the practice of disciplining the mind, body, and spirit to optimum capacity. It is the practice of mindfulness, compassion, grace, and love through all actions. If you are seeking enlightenment and bliss, for yourself and to share with others, I invite you to explore the magnitude of this philosophy so that you can come to learn, along with me, how to better our lives with its many teachings.

Namaste,
Christy

THE BIG PICTURE

WHY YOGA NOW?

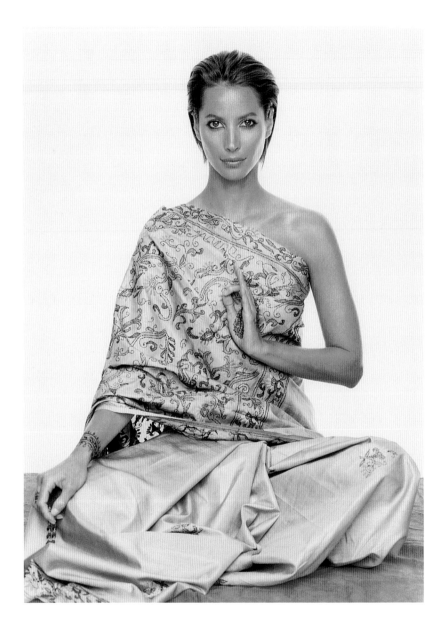

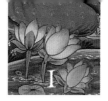

I

Today, people are turning to yoga for many reasons.

Those reasons range from managing one's stress to

preventative health measures, healing the body from

addictions, or perhaps simply because it is "trendy."

For some, it has been prescribed as therapy for an ail-

ment or injury, or it is the means to achieving a

desired physique—"the yoga body." The truth of the

matter is, yoga can and does serve many, if not all, of

these reasons, but the real purpose of this practice is

far from just physical. Physical strength may be developed, but the ultimate purpose of yoga is the inner journey, unique to each practitioner. In the beginning, a teacher may indeed be an important factor, and practicing in a group may provide a support that is absent when practicing alone, but eventually you will arrive at a place where you, and only you, can take yourself deeper. That is the point when you must go beyond your classes and discover what yoga is for you.

Many of us who are drawn to yoga share aspirations of freedom, but we soon realize the real journey to freedom begins inside. Once you start the journey, there is no return. This personal journey will require courage, as others may have a hard time accepting the changes you may choose as you find your way along on this quest. Once you discover yoga, however, you will feel empowered by the knowledge that you have cultivated and the necessary tools with which you have been equipped, especially the breath, which will bring you back home to yourself time and again. You may find, as I did, that the breath can be one of the greatest friends or lovers we will ever know. The breath is more intimate than anything else could ever be because it reaches the innermost spaces inside of our bodies. With the breath, we are never alone.

I have been a student of yoga myself since 1988, and have learned so much along the way, just as you have or will. I felt compelled to write *Living Yoga* as I looked around at the recent gain in popularity of the practice, both here and in the East. I felt that perhaps I could help other students like myself, who can so easily become overwhelmed or even misled by the vast information that is currently available. I felt that far too much misdirected attention was being brought to yoga for the wrong reasons, such as the emphasis on the outwardly physical benefits of the practice (a typical cultural obsession of we Westerners) or the publicity of celebrity endorsements, which seems to be more the fault of the media's fascination with us.

Whatever the causes, this explosion of enthusiasm and interest in yoga has also caused the yoga community to have some mixed feelings about this seemingly sudden growth. On the one hand, the exposure has brought about, for the first time, an enormous amount of global awareness about these practices. This is all exciting and good, but on the other hand, it has also encouraged many inexperienced practitioners to teach prematurely, which can result in causing unnecessary harm to curious beginners. Another problem is that, due to this rapidly-increasing popularity, there are now many overcrowded classrooms due to the demand outweighing the supply. And, without any realistic solution for standardizing yoga-teaching methods, which is not at all the most welcomed idea because of the innumerable forms and schools taught around the world, this can be dangerous territory to tread on.

Nonetheless, yoga is gaining more popularity, and more and more people of all walks are seeking information. It is my hope that this book will be a useful tool in guiding your questions to the appropriate resources, as well as

by showing, as an example, how valuable yoga has become to me in my daily life. This has been a challenging project, but one that has helped to solidify my understanding of the principles and teachings of yoga and reaffirm my personal path. As the saying goes, we often teach what we most need to learn ourselves, and in writing much of this book, I was reminded of all that I already knew and how much I need to listen to my own inner voice. With all of this knowledge that I currently hold and have recently gained, there is no reason for me to live in any way that does not serve me on my spiritual path. So, student to student, I share with you my experiential understanding of yoga in the following pages, as we are all connected by the common interest to discover the Self (your person on an exalted level; the level at which we connect with universal consciousness) on our journey of existence. Walk on.

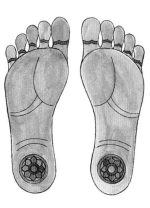

Symbols and Their Meanings

If we think of the letters of the alphabet as the basic building blocks to verbal expression, then we would have to consider symbols as the visual language of humanity. Since before the beginning of time, symbols have provided insights into understanding human nature. Whether they are precise depictions of recognizable reality or esoteric representations of the inner world, their roles are significant.

Throughout all of civilization, symbols have provided the power of communication in art, religion, ritual, and written text. They are a part of the many layers of our lives, from our intuition to our emotional and spiritual states. Within the context of spirituality and religion, and particularly here within the tradition of yoga, these symbols help to provide an added dimension to understanding the importance of the vocabulary and the history of yoga.

It is important to keep in mind, however, that when discussing symbols, their representations and meanings vary on a spectrum of many different cultural perspectives. According to Carl Jung (for further reading, see Jung, ed., *Man and His Symbols*, London: Arkana, 1990), a pioneering theorist on the meaning of symbols, symbolism is a part of a universal language and an integral part of understanding the psychic process. For Jung, archetypal symbols, for example, can be used to explore the conscious and unconscious mind and to better understand oneself. "The quest for self-knowledge through symbols is not the exclusive territory of Jungian psychology: to know oneself is an aspect of the enlightenment of which all the great philosophical and religious traditions speak," according to David Fontana's *The Secret Language of Symbols*.

In fact, the diversity in symbolic meaning extends far beyond Jung, and depends widely on the fact that the human mind is creatively limited and differs from person to person. Two people can offer very different interpretations of the same stimulus. Two cultures can either adapt or reinvent a symbol to accommodate their own belief system and iconography. Overall, symbols are subject to the passing of time, to the arrogance of intellectualization, to cultural commodification, and so forth. But they also have the potential to accumulate power over the ages and to evolve.

In this book, we look at those symbols most frequently associated with the subject at hand, as well as those symbols that offer evidentiary support for the universality of spirituality and the ability of yoga as life-practice to transcend religion. With this in mind, it is plain to see how symbols have enriched and continue to enrich the mind, the body, and the pursuit of learning.

Baddha Konasana (cover image)

When translated, *baddha* means "bound" or "caught," *kona* means "angle." With the knees bent at an acute angle out to the sides, the heels of the feet touching

each other near the perineum, and the feet caught by the hands, baddha konasana is a very important asana, especially when held for as long as possible. This posture is a particular blessing to women, as it tones the kidneys and alleviates urinary and uterine disorders, in addition to relieving menstrual discomfort and the symptoms of menopause. It helps prevent sciatica and hernia, and it strengthens the bladder and uterus. The posture also stretches the inner thighs, groin, and knees, and can even relieve depression and fatigue.

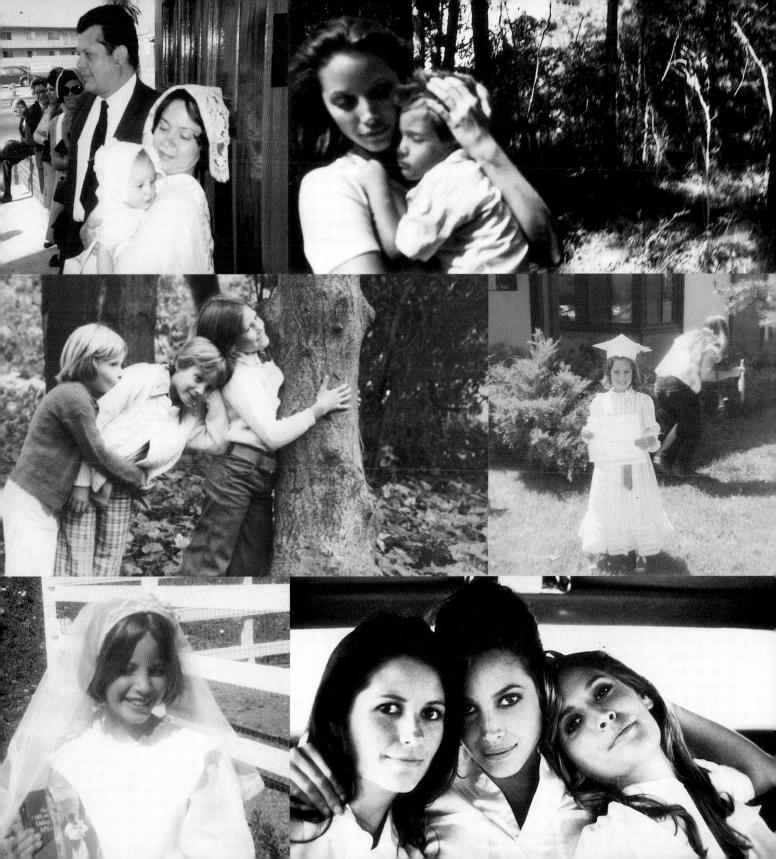

GRACE

"I do not understand the mystery of grace—only that it meets us where we are, but does not leave us where it found us."
—ANNE LAMOTT

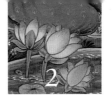

2

My sisters and I were born very closely to one another, all within the span of three years. For the most part, we have managed to stay close throughout our lives. When we were younger, we worked out a rotation plan that would allow us each to take a turn as the other's maid of honor, long before there were any prospects in line (although the birth order took a bit of a detour when my younger sister Erin married before me, the middle daughter).

My older sister, Kelly, was first. She married at twenty-six, and produced my parents' first grandchild a year later. I was in Paris for the spring collections when her baby son was born. I had dreamt of his arrival the previous night, then amazingly awoke to a phone call from my mom in California telling me the exciting news and details of his birth. They named him James, after his father.

His given name aside, we have called him so many things. My dad would call him Tinker, much to our collective dismay, because someone had given him that name when he was a boy. Because he was first, he was our little guinea pig of sorts. He was also the first of a new generation in our family full of girls. He seemed to give each of us something back— something buried deep inside of our hearts that rose to the surface and allowed us to love and feel loved in a new way. Everything we gave seemed to bounce right back from him, and we were genuinely happy when he was near. He was the object and subject of everything, and it was he, this tiny and helpless creature, who truly made us feel like a unified family again.

Since I was a teenager, I have always had to travel a lot because of my job, and as a result, had missed many important family events. Not just any events, but big ones—like Kelly's college graduation, Erin's graduation from high school, various family members' weddings, showers, and the like. My sisters once put together a photo album of themselves during those years when I first began to work as a model. When I look at it, it makes me sad to see how much they did together that I missed out on, as we all matured from girls into women.

Perhaps that's why I often found myself seeking some sense of comfort in unexpected places. For instance, when I traveled as a young woman, I would always go out of my way to visit churches—sometimes just to light a candle for someone in my prayers. I found solace in the sheer beauty of the architecture, the incense at a high mass, and the silence that embraces you when you enter a sacred space. My religious background was not enough to provide me with a constant sense of guilt, but as I got older, it did give me enough faith to ensure that I never would feel completely alone.

As I matured, I was aware of the obvious discord between the position of the Catholic church, in particular, and the reality of the times in which we were living. Here I was, a teenager in the midst of the 1980s, working in a business where hundreds of colleagues and friends were dying of AIDS. The church I believed I "belonged to" was officially opposed to same-sex relationships. I wondered, where did this leave their souls then? What if they had been baptized? Wasn't that supposed to be regarded as insurance in some way?

These may seem like strange questions, but it was my baptism that connected me to the Catholic church in the first place, and also what drew me into those sacred spaces across Europe. I had yet to really examine my faith, yet I still felt welcome to participate no matter where I was in the world, because I was already a member. And, while belonging mattered to me, I remained conflicted. I wasn't in agreement with everything the church said, and I didn't know where that left me, either. I still had much to explore.

When I was asked to be James's godmother, I was deeply touched because it immediately brought me closer to my spirituality than when I was merely an aunt. It also established a spir-itual bond between James and me. This was the first major commitment I had ever been invit-ed to take on, so I chose to take it very seri-ously, deservedly so. As godmother, my role was to become a spiritual guide to my nephew. In order to be a guide of this magnitude, I needed to resolve my relationship to the church and renew my commitment and faith. At twenty-five years of age, I viewed this as an opportuni-ty to explore my spirituality further.

After this cathartic rebirth that I was experi-encing after James's birth, I decided to go back to school the following year. I had been swept up by my career at the age of fifteen, and hadn't really stopped to catch my breath in over ten years. I longed to feel settled, and I craved a routine. I also wanted my life to have a purpose and to mean something. I felt that by returning to school, I would also come to know more of myself. I applied to NYU in the summer of 1995 for the fall semester. I started out part-time because I was unsure of what I would be able to handle. I never really loved school as a child, and had begun to work at such a young age that high school didn't stand a chance of rivaling the experiences of an adventurous and precocious young woman like myself. But I was now in a position of financial security, which allowed me the luxury of an adult education at a private university. I continued to work as a model for a few loyal clients as I eased into my new life, but for the most part, I was playing the role of a student now.

The same year that I entered school, I celebrated a victory over my longtime addiction to cigarettes. Perhaps it had come partly because I had gained a renewed appreciation for the miracle of life when James was born. I had started smoking at thirteen years old, and had spent the last seven years struggling to quit. I was gaining more self-respect as I came into womanhood, and smoking no longer fit with what I was committed to cultivating in myself. The act itself seemed to contradict my new role as a godmother, too. I now had an added responsibility, and owed it to myself and to my godson to live an exemplary and long life, thus making a healthier lifestyle a priority. Quitting smoking would affect my career, too, but it would also expedite an inevitable transition that I was more than ready for.

Soon after quitting smoking, I decided to eliminate other unhealthy activities as well, including the grueling lifestyle associated with runway modeling. After making this lifestyle change, I sought a routine, and went about creating one for myself. I was searching for mental and spiritual stimulation that my work could never afford me. I now had classes two days a week, and regularly attended church each Sunday. At school I had started off with basic requirements, but soon became a full-time student by the spring, adding art history and some interdisciplinary courses to my schedule. I also purchased an old town house close to campus in Greenwich Village, which was in dire need of refurbishing.

I moved in the following fall, just in time for my family's favorite holiday, Thanksgiving. My house was large enough to hold my entire family, all under one roof, and so I insisted on a New York reunion. My parents arrived early to help unpack the dishware and the books in the library, and help me prepare for the others. I had designed the layout for the purposes of holidays and frequent family get-togethers in New York. Each of my sisters now had a child of her own (Erin's daughter, Greer, was born earlier that spring). My grandmother came along, too. We enjoyed a near-perfect holiday. All together for the first time in my adopted city, we christened my new home. That would be my father's last

Thanksgiving, and each year when it comes around, I am thankful that we were able to share it.

Now that I had a "real" home, I joined a local parish—St. Joseph's, just a few blocks away. I went to mass in several nearby churches before choosing St. Joseph's. It's a small Greek revival style building, reportedly the oldest Catholic church still standing in Manhattan. The clergy consists of three priests, Fathers Tos, Laferty, and Halloran, and one nun, Sister Anne Tahaney. A small red-freckled woman with bright eyes, always smiling or winking at me from the dais, she, along with her sister, also a nun, had spent the better part of their religious careers in Pakistan. What immediately impressed me about this congregation was the diversity of its parishioners, the general aesthetic of the masses, and the fact that each member was known by name. Mass became a weekend break from my studies, and an opportunity to bask in gratitude.

Shortly after Christmas, that same year, my dad was diagnosed with lung cancer. Since he was a lifelong smoker, this was no surprise. Prayer became an even more essential part of my day. In the difficult months that followed, my faith, my routine classes, and my focus in school offered a refuge from the reality we were facing—that my father would inevitably die.

My father's death six months later had an enormous impact on every aspect of my life. When you lose someone so close to you, you lose a part of yourself, too. My relationship with my dad suddenly felt very close, as I had always looked up to him and strived toward his ideals. I realized I had to begin to reevaluate my other relationships, too. I had not gotten a lot of support from my partner throughout this challenging time, and it inevitably made me question why I was choosing to stay in the relationship. It was the only thing in my life holding me back . . . and I wanted to move forward. I decided to take some time for myself and go to a small holistic cleansing center down in Palm Springs that I'd heard people talking about at work. It was summer and school was out, so I flew to California, rented a car, and set out for the desert to contemplate my life and mourn my loss.

I arrived at We Care around lunchtime (though there was no lunch to be had). I went through an orientation and was given a week's supply of herbs and a schedule, and shown to my modest room. There was a strict regime of herbs and drinks designed to detoxify the body and restore health to the stressed out and the ill. Each day would begin at 6:00 A.M. with a brisk walk, followed by a gentle yoga class just before nutrition classes, lymphatic massages, and colonics. The rest of the days were spent reading and writing in my journal. Occasionally I rented some of their health and nutrition videos.

The basic premise of their program is based on the idea that disease begins internally, and can be prevented with proper nutrition and regular cleansing to remove the waste matter that can become lodged in the intestines and become harmful when they release streams of toxins into the body. Every day we fill our bodies with all sorts of chemicals, and we are not given enough time to process them entirely. This affects everything from how we feel emotionally to how we think, and, subsequently, how much energy we have throughout the day. In my opinion, the best medicine is preventative, which comes in a variety of ways (regular exercise, a balanced diet, a mindful lifestyle). I left We Care feeling clear-minded and revitalized. I had vowed to make a healthier lifestyle a priority. And thus far, I was

doing it. I promised myself to continue with yoga, which I'd rediscovered, when I got back home, and to pay more attention to what I would put into my body from that point on.

My father was as much an example in dying as he was in life, and I returned to New York in September with yet another renewed commitment to myself—I would return to a regular yoga practice. I vividly remember my first yoga class at Jivamukti in the East Village. My good friend Prema brought me with her one afternoon after school. The class was on the first floor of a walk-up on Third Avenue in the East Village. The center was small and packed full with students. The class was taught by someone who would become one of my future teachers, Sharon Gannon. It had been some time since my last serious yoga class, and this was my first in New York City. Her gentle voice immediately brought me back to my earliest connection to Kundalini Yoga, and the classes I had attended in California some years before.

I followed along with the other students in *vinyasa*, until we reached the final series of inversions. The poses were familiar, but not the pace. Prema and I were in the center of the long, narrow, lavender painted room, which had grown warm and sticky from the perspiration of so many jammed together. When everyone went into the commanded headstand pose, I joined the others, as if I had assumed the posture only yesterday. Just as I managed to balance my legs directly above me, Sharon walked by. At that moment, I had been thinking about what I must have looked like from an outside perspective, so tall and lanky, when I fell, my legs crashing down, barely missing the yogi behind me. I landed with a bang, my lower back hitting one of the wooden blocks that were designed to assist you in the more difficult poses. But despite my tumble, I wasn't fazed. I felt so good walking out of the door from class that I knew I would be back.

As my lifestyle was changing, so, too, was my focus in school. My courses changed, as well, reflecting the influence of the last several months. I enrolled in classes called "Death and Dying," "Theism, Atheism, and Existentialism," and "Jungian Dream Analysis." The last greatly appealed to me, as I had been having numerous dreams about my father since his passing. I was a junior now, and it was becoming clear that my academic concentration was being redirected toward the spiritual. Somehow, I felt closer to my dad than ever, as our separation was no longer a matter of mere mileage. He was here with me now, whenever and however I needed him to be. I felt comforted by his regular visits to my subconscious. Though he was much the same dad, in my dreams he always appeared frailer than he had been physically in real life, and he maintained this final weakened state in my dreams for a long time.

With my new commitment to yoga and my current studies, I couldn't help but feel compelled to do something more with my loss; to create something from the absence. With the advice of a friend, I contacted several health organizations to join the effort in helping others fight their addictions to tobacco. The Centers for Disease Control and Prevention took me up on my offer, and we were soon ready to film a public service announcement. That was in January of 1998. I had worked with an advertising agency in Massachusetts to create a message for their "Truth" series. The collaboration was a success, and the PSA is still running today, nearly five years after my dad's death. This would be the beginning of a personal crusade, one that commemorated my father's life and one, like yoga, that could celebrate all of ours.

THE ORIGINS OF YOGA

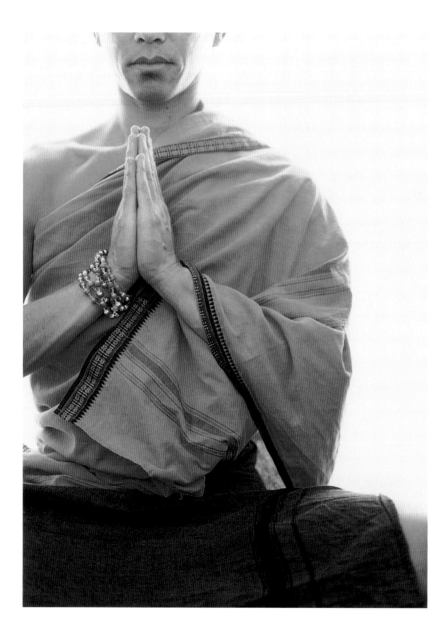

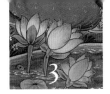

3

It is impossible to assign one definition to yoga . . . as impossible, in fact, as it would be to assign one definition to God. For example, our Western *Webster's* dictionary defines yoga as follows: (1) A series of postures and breathing exercises practiced to attain physical and mental control and tranquility; (2) A school of Hindu philosophy using yoga to unify the self with the Supreme Being. Though the Sanskrit word *yoga* does indeed translate to "union" or

Sanskrit

Sanskrit is the sacred language of India. Sanskrit was the language of the learned and upper classes of India, in which most literature and philosophical works were written. The oldest form of Sanskrit is the language of the Vedic hymns, and was later codified by the yogi Panini in 500 B.C.E. Sanskrit continued as the language of the scholarly and holy even after the language itself had evolved and split into regional vernaculars. A "natural" language, Sanskrit represents the fundamental tones and sounds of nature and the world itself, and thus resonates these vibrations in its spoken form. Literally translated, Sanskrit means "perfectly constructed speech." Because of the crucial role that sound plays in the Hindu tradition and in the practices of yoga, Sanskrit is the language in which mantras and relevant sacred scripts are written and spoken. It is also the language of the true names of the asanas.

"to yoke or harness," as in yoking with and uniting the mind and body or the individual and universal consciousness, what it is we commune with and the means by which we do so vary across many sources, teachers, and practices.

In one sense of the word, yoga refers to that vast body of spiritual beliefs, physical techniques, and scholarly philosophy first developed in India over 5,000 years ago. On another generic level, yoga is the name applied to numerous spiritual paths of transcendence and liberation from the self and the ego. The application of the term yoga, the tradition of which, in fact, predates religion of any kind, has even been extended to other traditions that have clearly been influenced throughout history by the original Indian source of inspiration. Tibetan Yoga (*Vajrayana Buddhism*),

Japanese "Yoga" (*Zen*), and Chinese "Yoga" (*Cha'an*) all share similarities in philosophy and practice with Indian Yoga. From certain angles, yoga even overlaps with aspects of Judaism and Christianity. Though they all developed quite independently of one another, Judaism and Christianity have traditions of mysticism and transcendence, particularly within their traditions of ritual, just as in yoga. Also, especially with the rise in popularity of yoga in the West in the last half of this century, many parallels can be drawn between all of these spiritual practices.

On one spiritual level, yoga refers to the union of the Individual Self with the Universal Self. For other believers, it may be better understood as a union of the physical, physiological, mental, emotional, and intellectual bodies, leading its practitioners to live an integrated, purposeful, useful, and noble life. Of course, I am not the first to say that yoga is so much more. I can only try my best to guide you through what I have learned through my studies at University and—perhaps even more importantly—through the knowledge I have gained in my own personal practice and exploration of a spiritual path. I will do my best to guide you through the many options that this ancient philosophy has to offer. I am merely a student myself, seeking a way that will allow me to explore as many paths as I possibly can within this lifetime.

As we have evolved and continue to evolve, yoga, too, has, over time, continued to branch and evolve such that assigning it succinct meaning makes it easier to begin to appreciate just how great the tradition is and how universal the practices can still be today. Throughout the history of yoga, various texts have ascribed to it many different meanings. Patanjali's *Yoga Sutras*, which present the eight limbs of yoga and which we will explore further in this book, emphasize the restraint of the mind and the coming in contact with the transcendental Self through focusing the entire body. According to the *Bhagavad Gita*, considered to be one of the most powerful works on yoga in the form of an epic poem, yoga is "skill in action" and "equanimity" or "balance." Yoga aims to purify the mind and body. It is an ethical discipline and offers a way

The Hindu Pantheon

Part of yoga's universal appeal, to both Easterners and Westerners, is its vast adaptability to all people and lifestyles regardless of religious upbringing or spiritual state. Taken at face value, yoga is a wonderful tool for maintaining and cultivating one's physical health. As we know, however, its tradition and depth is far, far greater. And though yoga differs—through its many schools, meditation styles, and philosophical variances—among its many traditions, it is important to recognize its vital connection to Hindu cosmology, especially as it is so frequently referenced in this book. Regardless of your own spiritual practice, whether it be monotheistic or polytheistic, Eastern or Western, part of the beauty of the yoga tradition lies in the intricacies of its rich legendary fabric.

There are several major deities that are worshiped as the Supreme Being in the Hindu tradition. Some practitioners regard Shiva as the ultimate divine manifestation. Others see the god Vishnu as the Supreme. Others still worship more specifically certain manifestations or incarnations of deities who each represent aspects of characteristics of Brahman, the indescribable supreme being, known to many of us as God. For example, Vaishnavites (devotees of Vishnu) are devoted to Krishna, one of the many incarnations of Vishnu. Regardless, worshipers have focused on various distinguishing features of Vishnu. Since the very early roots of Hinduism, deities have been largely perceived through three main characteristic groups—their material, psychological, and spiritual symbolism.

One god of particular interest is Shiva, pictured here as the "Lord of the Dance." The *Rig Veda*, a collection of very early hymns composed around 1500 B.C.E., includes mentions of Shiva, a god of ambiguity and inconsistency, and also the three-eyed god—his eyes represent the sun, moon, and fire, and reveal all that is of the past, present, and future—with a crescent moon, symbolizing knowledge and mystical vision, in his wild, matted hair. He embodies opposites, is both male and female, and one glance from the third eye situated in the middle of the forehead is powerful enough to incinerate the universe. Around Shiva's neck, the *kundalini*, or serpent energy of the *shakti*, located in the spine, is coiled.

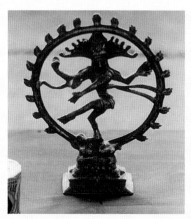

Sometimes, Shiva is considered a god of destruction, though to his worshipers he is the great creator and maintainer, as well as destroyer, of the cosmos. He is iconographically portrayed most commonly as the Lord of Yoga, meditating in the Himalayas, with the Ganges River cascading from the crown of his head; as a family man with his goddess wife, Parvati, their sons, Skanda and Ganesha, and the bull Nandin, a sacred symbol of sexual energy; as the four-armed Lord of the Dance, cosmic creator and destroyer, dancing on the "dwarf of ignorance" surrounded by a circle of flames; and as Shiva *linga* seen with the linga, a representation of a phallus within a vulva, meant to represent the male and female creativity and the union of Shiva with his

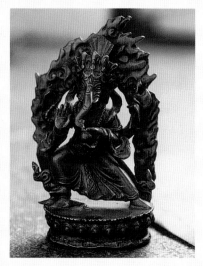

shakti. Shiva is more widely considered part of the Hindu creation "trinity." Shiva's son Ganesha, the elephant-headed deity, also called "Lord of the Hosts," comes up frequently in Hindu iconography and is worshiped as a remover of spiritual obstacles.

Like Shiva, Vishnu ("Pervader") is mentioned early on in the Rig Veda. Hindu mythology places Vishnu at the creation of the world when he takes three strides and separates the earth from the sky. Vishnu is very often depicted as a dark blue youth with four arms, representing omnipresence and omnipotence, each holding his distinguishing elements—a conch (creation), a discus (universal mind), a mace (life force), and a lotus (the universe). He possesses a lock of golden hair on his chest that symbolizes the core of nature. Another depiction is of Vishnu resting on the coils of the cosmic serpent Shesa, or Ananta, floating on the infinite cosmic ocean of formless existence. Vaishnavites believe that he is the transcendent Lord who dwells in the highest heaven but manifests himself in the world in order to restore *dharma* (virtue) in times of darkness. He is believed to have manifested himself in ten incarnations (*avatara*) thus far, as Matsya (Fish), Kurma (Tortoise), Varaha (Boar), Narasimha (Man-Lion), Vamana (Dwarf), Parashurama (Rama with the Axe), Rama or Ramacandra ("Dark One" or "Pleasing One"), Krishna ("Puller," a God-man), Buddha ("Awakened One"), and Kalki ("Base One"), who is yet to come. These incarnations focus on the many aspects of creation, destruction, and recreation of the cosmic universe.

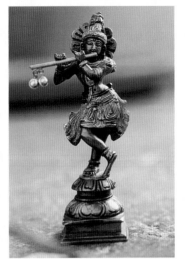

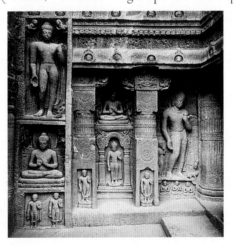

While both Vishnu and Shiva are the most iconographically revered and depicted deities within Hindu spirituality, there is certainly a strong and essential goddess-worship tradition as well. Many of the goddesses are venerated as manifestations or facets of Maha Devi, the Great Goddess. Often contradictory, the Hindu goddess can be treated as a benevolent and nurturing mother figure, as well as a spiteful and demanding force. While most goddesses, such as Lakshmi, Lalita Tripura-Sundari, Durga, and Sarasvati, have groups of worshipers devoted specifically to them, nearly all are revered to some extent by Hindus. Lakshmi is the goddess of beauty and adornment, for instance; each has a specific purpose.

of living life neutrally, exercising modesty, and experiencing as a result a freedom from pain and sorrow.

Just as the word *yoga* can mean so many things in ancient scriptures and to modern scholars, the yogi herself can explore all of the facets of this tradition, and through them discover the path that is right for her. And although yoga is indeed a spiritual path and one based on ancient sacred philosophy that originated in India, it is not necessary to ascribe to any particular religious tradition. Yoga is so universal in its principles and so holistically beneficial, it is possible for any person, young or old, religious or agnostic, to embrace and enjoy a practice.

IN ORDER TO learn about what yoga truly is, it's important to know some of the historic context around the word itself. In terms of Pre-Classical (approximately 1000–100 B.C.E., during which the earliest complete work of yoga, the Bhagavad Gita, is dated) and Post-Classical schools of yoga (roughly from the seventh to seventeenth centuries, during which nondualistic—meaning no separation between transcendental Self and the transcendental Reality or Absolute—thinking nurtured traditions like Hatha Yoga), the basic idea of yoga as a union with the Absolute is perfectly adaptable. However, the Classical school of yoga, greatly defined by Patanjali's Yoga Sutras (perhaps the most authoritative text on yoga), defines yoga as a focusing of the attention "to whatever object is being contemplated to the exclusion of all others" (as stated by Georg Feuerstein in *The Yoga Tradition*). But first, let's look at its beginnings.

For many centuries, it was believed that yoga arrived with the Aryan invasion, along with all other aspects of advanced Indian culture, around 1500 B.C.E. The Aryans came from ancient central Asia and were a tall, light-skinned, Sanskrit-speaking people who are credited with important elements of India's heritage of spiritual civilization, religious, social, and economic institutions. While bringing these elements, their warlike culture enabled them to dominate the darker-skinned indigenous Indians, whose literary and

Yoga Timeline

Indus Valley Civilization	2500 B.C.E.–1500 B.C.E.
Vedic period begins	1500 B.C.E.
Rig Veda revealed	1500 B.C.E.–1200 B.C.E.
Flourishing of the Vedas	1200 B.C.E.–500 B.C.E.
The Buddha b. Prince Siddhartha Gautama	600 B.C.E.–500 B.C.E.
Upanishads written, end of the Veda	600 B.C.E.–300 B.C.E.
Sanskrit codified by Panini	500 B.C.E.
The Mahabarata (with the Bhagavad Gita) is written. Major developments: theism—movement of devotional faith in development of Patanjali's (Yoga Sutras) Hindu deities, especially Vishnu, Shiva, and Devi	500 B.C.E.–300 B.C.E.
Patanjali's Yoga Sutras written, probably around 200 B.C.E.	200 B.C.E.–800 C.E.

philosophical traditions had evolved long before, as proven by the discovery of the Indus Valley civilization, a highly developed culture existing at least two thousand years earlier than the Aryans. The findings of these excavations in the first half of the twentieth century indicate the pre-Aryan beginnings of worship of Shiva and also of the Mother Goddess, which leads to the current view that Hinduism probably originated in India, intersecting with Aryan culture through creating the Vedas and Vedanta. Among the artwork that was found were intricate carvings of Shiva sitting in *mulabandhasana,* one of the most demanding yoga postures, which depicts Yogic mastery.

A more accurate description of yoga than that provided by *Webster's* would be that it is one of the six systems of Indian philosophy. At first, yoga was communicated orally over many generations, like many other cultures and spiritual practices around the world. Yogic history became more precise when the two great yoga texts were first written down. The Bhagavad Gita, which is part of the *Mahabharata* epic, is credited to the sage Vyasa and dated closer to the fifth century B.C.E. Then, sometime between the fifth and second century B.C.E., the Indian sage Patanjali compiled the *Yoga Darshana,* more commonly known today as the Yoga Sutras of Patanjali, though both Vyasa and Patanjali are considered to be more the "assemblers" of an existing oral tradition than actual authors. The Bhagavad Gita praises yoga and illustrates the divine relationship between mortals and Supreme Consciousness, while the Yoga Sutras provide practical instructions on how to achieve its promises. The latter text forms the basis of yoga philosophy as we know it today.

When we enter further into the world of yoga and the physical postures, called *asanas,* you may be overwhelmed by the many names that get thrown around in classes, and you may find it initially difficult to get your bearings. Many of those names will be difficult to remember, let alone pronounce. Personally, I always find that reading and telling stories is the best way to remember individuals' lives, especially when they feel so remote to our own. Yoga is very much a handed down tradition, and it is important to understand how it has come to you, here and now. There are innumerable men and women, gurus, writers, holy persons, scholars, and enthusiasts who have all contributed to the development and evolution of contemporary yoga—so innumerable, in fact, that it would take at least an entire book to just begin to honor them. Here, however, are a few important stories about some of the founding fathers of yoga as we have come to know it today.

The Vedas, Upanishads, and Vedanta

The history of yoga reaches as far back as the Vedic period, which began about 1500 B.C.E. This period of significant cultural development left behind a crucial legacy of literary contributions that formed the philosophical and spiritual roots for the development of Hinduism. The collection of scriptures left behind by the people of the Vedic age are known as the *Vedas*. The Vedas are classified into four categories according to content and chronology. The first category, *Samhita*, is a collection of four hymns—the *Rig Veda*, *Yajur Veda*, *Sama Veda*, and *Atharva Veda*—with the Rig Veda considered the oldest and most significant collection of hymns, comprising the heart of Vedic philosophy.

The second category, *Brahmanas*, was largely prose interpretations of the older texts and helped clarify the essence of the Vedic beliefs and practices. Third were the *Aranyakas*, which took a close look at the submerged symbolism within the rituals outlined in the previous collections. The fourth and later the most significant category of the Vedas are the *Upanishads*.

The collection of scriptures as a whole comprises what has become the basic textual (though they were transmitted orally for centuries) foundation for the Hindu belief system. Many people are inclined to compare Indian belief in the Vedas to what the Torah, New Testament, or the Koran means to Jews, Christians, and Muslims. Like these Western sacred texts, parts of which are believed to express divine truth as it was directly communicated by God, the Vedic Samhitas are the records of divine truth as it was revealed by God to the great *rishis*, or saints, of ancient time.

Coming at the end of the Vedic age, an important time in the evolution of Hindu thinking, were the Upanishads. The mystical and somewhat radical teachings of the Upanishads laid the foundation for various yogic perspectives on core concepts such as the supreme *Brahman* (God) and *atman* (the self), *karma* (action) and *moksha* (liberation), and the liberation through *dhyana* (meditation) and *jnana* (knowledge), which all later further developed into the discipline of yoga. As they were the last installation in the Vedas, but still considered part of the divine truth as revealed through scripture—as opposed to later teachings that were considered "tradition" by comparison—the Upanishad philosophical system is also called, appropriately, Vedanta ("the end of the Veda"). The Upanishads, and therefore of the classification Vedanta, encompass a vast body of some two hundred texts, and span hundreds of years. However, only a small portion of these writings date back, in their orally-transmitted form, to Vedic times.

One of the most important yoga texts ever to be recorded was the Bhagavad Gita, part of a larger body of work called the Mahabharata, which is considered an Upanishad because of certain trademark elements. The Bhagavad Gita is usually dated between the third and fifth centuries B.C.E., a time during which "theism"—the concept of devotion to a particular deity that grew into a major aspect of Hinduism—became popular. Two deities that were most widely focused on were Vishnu and Shiva. While there are few texts of such magnitude dedicated to Shiva, the Bhagavad Gita represents a monumental sacred work about Lord Krishna, an incarnation of the god Vishnu. The Bhagavad Gita translates as "Song of the Lord," and is the earliest extant document of Vaishnavism, the religion devoted to the worship of Vishnu, specifically as Krishna, and one of the major religions in India. The Bhagavad Gita's teachings of the eternal love between Divinity and devotees, as well as its communication of Krishna's visions on how to achieve peace and enlightenment, are integral to contemporary yoga practice and continue to provide inspirations of the ideal to people of all spiritual and philosophical walks of life. The main themes of the Gita, as it is often referred to, are the importance of dharma (religious duty), the importance of non-attachment and karma, that the soul is immortal, and that the Lord is reached through *bhakti* (devotion) and by his grace.

Yoga's Founding Fathers

PATANJALI, THE YOGA SUTRAS, AND THE EIGHT LIMBS

Patanjali's Yoga Sutras ("threads") is a text that covers many aspects of life, beginning with a code of conduct and ending with a man's vision of his true self to illustrate the path and goal of yoga to the reader. Like the Buddhist Eightfold Path, this yogic path, made up also of eight steps, offers a method of awakening; a course in which higher consciousness can be attained. The eight aspects, or *astanga* (limbs), of yoga are the *yamas, niyamas, asanas, pranayama, pratyahara, dharana, dhyana,* and *samadhi.* The yamas and niyamas are codes of moral and social conduct. The yamas are comprised of consideration toward all living things, and the ability to communicate with sensitivity, non-violence, moderation in all our actions, and non-greediness. The niyamas comprise cleanliness, contentment, the removal of impurities in the mind and body, study and reverence to a higher intelligence, or the acceptance of our limitations in relation to God. In the asanas, one gains the dual qualities of alertness and relaxation without tension. These qualities, achieved by recognizing and observing the reactions of the body and breath to various postures, can help an individual endure and even minimize the external influences on the body, such as climate, diet, and work. They are also a way to reduce physical *avidya* (misunderstanding), because the body is an expression of the mind and its misapprehensions. In addition, asana practice also teaches us about the breath and how it behaves.

Pranayama, the restraint and control of one's breath, helps to reduce the obstacles that inhibit clear perception through breathing techniques. Pratyahara is the relaxation and internalization of the senses of perception, and occurs when the mind is able to remain in its chosen direction without distraction. Dharana, or concentration, is the ability to direct the mind toward a chosen object, in spite of many other potential objects within reach. Dhyana, or meditation, is the ability to develop focused interactions with what we seek to understand, and samadhi is the ultimate state of Self-realization, union with the source.

Yama, niyama, asana, and pranayama are considered *bahira sadhana* (external practices or studies), which can be taught by another. The first two limbs, especially, establish a wholesome and ethically correct way of life for the yogi. The third limb, asana, translates this into exercises for the body. Pratyahara and dharana are *antaranga sadhana* (internal practices), which are experiential states that cannot be taught and must be experienced individually. Dhyana and samadhi are *antaratma sadhanas* (studies concerning the innermost practices), in which one reaches an ecstatic supreme state, the ultimate state of self-realization. Though all of these limbs are essential to the yogic path of liberation, in this book I have chosen to explore only three in depth—asana, pranayama, and dhyana—as those are the three limbs that, for a majority of us, we will most frequently encounter and also need to reach the other states. The first two, yamas and niyamas, will come with regular practice. Pratyahara, dharana, and samadhi may also come from extended or concentrated practice.

Over time, numerous translations and commentaries have been written on these Yoga Sutras. Very little is known about the life of Patanjali, other than the fact that he is also credited with authorship of definitive texts on *Ayurveda,* the Indian system of medicine, and also on grammar. Many mythological images of Patanjali exist. He is often depicted as sheltered by a thousand-headed serpent with four hands, like Vishnu, holding a conch, a disk, a mace, and a sword; or as a half-man, half-serpent with a hood, upon which he carries the weight of the universe. At times, he also serves as the bed of Lord Vishnu. These two representations are intended to depict the perfected balance of yogic qualities—alert relaxation and irresistible stability in an asana.

Patanjali's Yoga Sutras, which were originally written in Sanskrit, the language of yoga, describe the nature and workings of the human mind, techniques to master the mind, and techniques to attain heightened and even superhuman capacities; as well as a path toward states of tranquility, happiness, and unlimited comprehension. The Sutras take their name from one of the many forms of Sanskrit literature, which consists of many forms, such as *shlokas, gadyas, puranas,* and *sutras.* Shlokas are executed as metrical couplets; gadyas are written in the form of prose. Puranas are epic tales such as the Mahabarata and Bhagavad Gita, rendered in both poetry and prose, while sutras are brief aphorisms with an exact and complex meaning that generates contemplation.

The Yoga Sutras total 195 of these aphorisms, which would traditionally have been taught and memorized as a chant. In one very famous sutra, Patanjali offers to us one of the earliest written definitions of yoga:

Yogashchittavrttinirodhah:

Yoga (union), *chitta* (mind), *vrtti* (activity), *nirodhah* (complete absorption).
"Yoga is the ability to direct the mind exclusively toward an object, and to sustain that direction without any distractions."
—PATANJALI'S YOGA SUTRAS

According to Patanjali's definition, as relayed in *Health, Healing & Beyond* by T. K. V. Desikachar, "Although 'object' can be a thing, it can also be 'anything' that the mind engages, including the furthest reaches of art, scientific knowledge, the cosmos, or, ultimately, God."

The Yoga Sutras are divided into four sections or chapters and, as in the four Gospels of the New Testament, are believed to be representations of the sage's teachings to four disciples, each at a different stage of Yogic development. The first chapter, called *Samadhi-pada,* or the chapter on samadhi, lays out the framework of yoga, its characteristics, the problems that will be encountered along the path, and how to deal with them, as well as the state of mind that results. Patanjali also tells us here that unbounded clarity and limitless intelligence, fulfilled as serenity and purity of action, are the true gifts of yoga.

In this crucial first chapter, Patanjali defines the mind as the activities that constitute it, and explains that all our perceptions of mind can only be in terms of five activities, which can be both problematic and beneficial. These five activities are: comprehension, misapprehension, imagination, deep sleep, and memory. He then offers some guidance about how to achieve a state of yoga, which he says can occur through practice and detachment. Practice is essentially a process of directed effort followed for a long time, without interruption, as a gradual progression. It is the backbone of all yoga, and it is also important that practice be conducted enthusiastically and with optimism to ensure success.

The second chapter is called *Sadhana-pada* (spiritual path), or the means by which we obtain the previously unobtainable. It teaches us that the practice of yoga will reduce both physical and mental impurities, develop our capacity for self-examination, and also help us

to understand that, ultimately, we are not the masters of everything that we do. Also in this chapter, Patanjali takes us to a deeper understanding of "misapprehension and its misdirection of our actions believed to be the source of all problems." This is what is known as *avidya*, or knowledge other than right knowledge. Avidya is the false state of understanding, which is when we think we are doing the right thing but it is inevitably wrong, or when we don't trust our instincts when we are right, and then convince ourselves otherwise.

In the third and final fourth chapters, *Vibhuti-pada* and *Kaivalya-pada*, Patanjali discusses the capacity of the mind to become free from distractions and deeply contemplative through the practices and concepts laid out in the first two sections. He points out that everything is relative, and achieving a deep concentration practice may come easily to one individual, but not to another. We must develop our capacities and through the practices (discipline, postures, breath, and sense control) we will gain ease over the control of our mind-body and achieve the highest state of yoga. Through this state we also gain an awareness of our actions, how they are influenced, and what they result in, as we simultaneously look inward at our mental qualities and gain new skills. Patanjali explores the clarity that the mind is capable of if we choose to seek it, and the vast potential thereof. Once we have reached the highest state of clarity, serenity will naturally flow in all of our actions as well as inactions.

Finally, in the Sutras, yoga teaches us that we are in fact infinitely more than our perceptions. The challenge is to develop the ability to discriminate between the perceiver within our selves and all that is outwardly perceived around us. Again, this can be accomplished through the mastery and practice of the eight limbs of yoga.

KRISHNAMACHARYA

Known as the premiere asana guru responsible for bringing yoga to the West, Tirumalai Krishnamacharya was born in November 1888 in Muchakundapuram, in the Karnataka state of India. Born a scholar and of the *Brahmin* (priestly) caste, he went to Mysore to study at the Parkala Math, a center of religious authority, disputation, learning, and law. At the age of thirteen, he went on to study at the University of Benares, also called Varanasi, considered the holiest of Indian cities among Hindus. While in Benares, Krishnamacharya practiced asanas and pranayama, which he had learned from his father, and was introduced to Sri Babu Bhagavan Das, a renowned yogi, who became his teacher at the nearby Patna University, before going on to study Vedanta.

Benares was founded as early as 3000 B.C.E. and is erected on the sacred Ganges River. Hindu pilgrims bathe along the river on the ghats to cleanse sins, and it is also believed that if you die there, you will go straight to heaven.

In 1915, Krishnamacharya set out on a Himalayan pilgrimage to Mount Kailash in Tibet, the eternal abode of Lord Shiva, where he met his next teacher, Sri Ramamohan, with whom he studied for the next seven years. His studies consisted of the philosophy and mental science of yoga, including the practice and perfection of asana and pranayama. In addition, he learned Patanjali's Yoga Sutras by heart, as well as how to chant them with perfection. He also cultivated some *siddhis,* or special powers, developed by practice, such as the ability to stop his own breath and heartbeat. Out of the supposed seven thousand asanas his teacher knew, Krishnamacharya is said to have mastered about three thousand. That is an astounding number considering that today, most serious or advanced students learn and teach only about fifty or sixty postures for their practices.

In 1931, Krishnamacharya received an invitation to teach at the Sanskrit College in Mysore, where the ruling family had fought to preserve many of the indigenous arts, including the *Sritattvanidhi,* perhaps the oldest illustrated asana compilations known. The Maharaja of Mysore helped Krishnamacharya to promote yoga throughout India for the next few decades through financially sponsoring asana demonstrations and tours. Then, when Krishnamacharya lost his post at the Sanskrit College, it was the maharaja who offered some space for a *yogashala,* or yoga school, in his palace for teaching. This is where Krishnamacharya developed and first taught what is now known as Astanga Vinyasa Yoga.

Eventually, Krishnamacharya divided the poses into three standardized sequences—primary, intermediate, and advanced—grouping students according to their ability, thus formulating his own school of yoga. During this period, he taught some of today's most renowned teachers, such as Sri K. Pattabhi Jois and B. K. S. Iyengar. Jois continues to teach Astanga Vinyasa Yoga in his guru's precise footsteps. Iyengar, also Krishnamacharya's brother-in-law, continues to teach a modified asana practice in Puna, India, today, which is considered more a healing and therapeutic type of asana practice.

In 1950, the yogashala was forced to close after India gained back her independence. Those who were chosen to replace the royal family of Mysore had little interest in asanas, but Krishnamacharya kept on teaching. In later years, his teaching techniques were said to have softened with his growing compassion, and he began to teach each individual to the best of his or her ability, similar to the technique that Iyengar uses today—he would vary the length, frequency, and sequencing of asanas to help students achieve more specific and short-term goals.

Astanga Vinyasa Yoga, as taught by Krishnamacharya, consists of five basic elements. The first involves asana, the physical postures of yoga. The second is pranayama, controlled breathing techniques. The third is chanting, which has a healing effect on the mind and body, and brings one into contact with the ancient and sacred language of Sanskrit. The fourth is dyhana meditation, which creates awareness both inward and outward beyond our usual mental limits. The fifth is ritual, an instinctive and universal human act. While ritual and chanting are key elements within the greater practice of yoga and in specific spiritual practices the world over, asana, pranayama, and meditation—three of the eight limbs of yoga—are those familiar essentials that I have chosen to explore here in depth and that I hope to make accessible to all practitioners, no matter what it is that you seek. Remember, you are that which you seek.

Baddha Padmasana
(bound lotus)

In this asana, the arms are crossed behind the back with the legs crossed in front and the toes caught by the hands. This posture opens the chest fully, making breathing much easier. The thyroids are massaged and the spinal column is stretched, as well as the waist, abdomen, and pelvis.

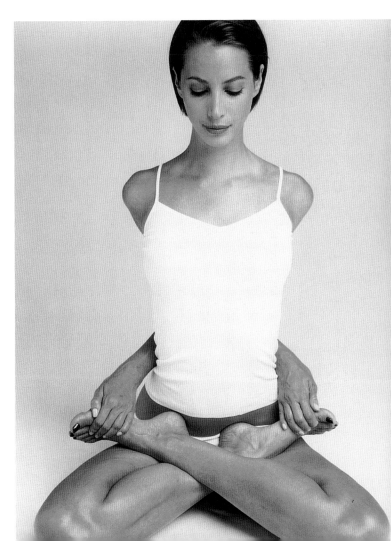

ASANAS (POSTURES)

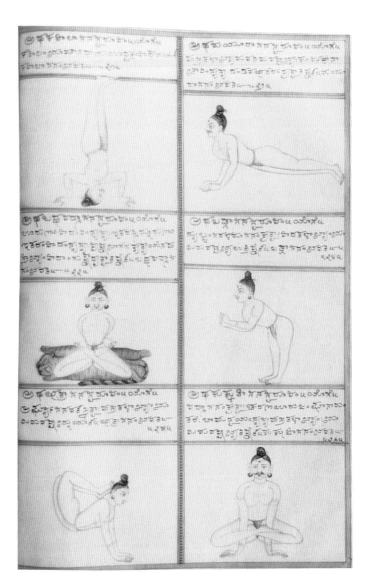

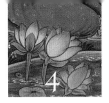

4

Many people in the West tend to think that yoga is a

single practice of physical postures, known as asanas,

but, as I mentioned earlier, there are in fact eight

forms or limbs (astanga) in total. The path of

Astanga Yoga incorporates each of these limbs as they

were designed, to help individuals reach the ultimate

limb, samadhi; the state of enlightenment or bliss.

The Sanskrit word *asana* means "seat." Literally, an

asana is a posture or a seated connection through

which a relationship to the earth is established. An asana practice is only spiritually enhanced when combined with other yoga practices, like pranayama and dhyana.

All asanas are actually part of a system called Hatha Yoga ("Ha" meaning "sun," "Tha" meaning "moon"), which refers to a vast area of doctrines and practices concerned with harnessing the *prana,* or life-force energy, that circulates throughout the human body. The meaning of the word itself conveys the intention of bringing two worlds of opposition together. It is a physical practice toward a spiritual goal. In fact, it is *the* physical practice of yoga. This body-oriented approach to transcendence involves cleansing practices, which include postures and breath control. (You may be wondering to yourself at this moment, what is the difference, then, between Hatha and Astanga? The truth is, Astanga Yoga is a part, or a school, of Hatha Yoga, which we will explore shortly.)

In the practice of asanas, we are using the body as a tool to shape ourselves for the experience of union with our higher or supreme consciousness. Not to mention the fact that the health benefits of the asana practices are innumerable. Through the twisting of the body and focused breathing during the practice, the internal organs and bloodstream are cleansed and purified, which can have a transforming effect on our general health while at the same time helping to prepare the body for a meditation practice. Creating energy movement within the body through physical movement assists in the calming or quieting of our minds so that we can connect with our innermost selves, each of which is intrinsically linked to creation. In the West, the asanas are often the entry point to yoga, which, over time, can lead a dedicated practitioner to greater awareness of his self and environment. A regular asana practice can also open the door to all the rest that the philosophy has to offer.

Today, there are several schools of asana, all of which stem from the Hatha Yoga tradition. Because so many of these schools are spin-offs of others, and because there are so many of them, it would be impossible and unnecessary to cover them all for the purposes of this book. Instead, I will explain the three most popular schools of yoga—Astanga Vinyasa Yoga, Iyengar Yoga, and Kundalini Yoga, all of which I have had personal experience with—and suggest resources for furthering your knowledge at your own pace. I will also briefly touch upon some of the other schools that have developed from them.

Astanga Vinyasa Yoga

Astanga Yoga, as taught by Sri K. Pattabhi Jois, began with the rediscovery, early in this century, of the *Yoga Korunta*. The Yoga Korunta is an ancient manuscript that describes a unique system of Hatha Yoga as practiced and created by the ancient sage Vamana Rishi. Pattabhi Jois is himself a renowned Sanskrit scholar and yogi, still living and teaching today in his late eighties in Mysore, India. Under the direction of his own guru, Krishnamacharya, this system of yoga was established and named Astanga Vinyasa Yoga, taking its name from the eight limbs, as both believed it to be the original asana practice intended by Patanjali.

The Yoga Korunta emphasizes vinyasa, or breath-synchronized movement, as a method of syn-chronizing progressive series of postures with a specific breathing technique. This technique is called *ujayyi pranayama* ("the victorious breath"), a process producing intense internal heat and a profuse sweat that purifies and detoxifies muscles and organs, which is used to enrich prana. The result is improved circulation, a light and strong body, and a calm mind. The basic premise for Astanga Vinyasa Yoga is to incorporate a posture sequence (there are six sequences total within this tradition) with the specific vinyasa breath-flow. This, in turn, flows from one level to the next, just as the path is laid out as the eight limbs in the Yoga Sutras: Movement through postures (asanas) purifies the physical body, while mastery and refine-ment of the breath (pranaya-

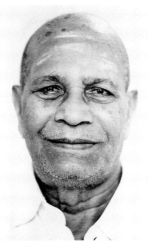
SRI K. PATTABHI JOIS

ma) through concentration (dharana) quiets the senses (pratyahara), preparing the practitioner for meditation (dhyana) and eventually the union of the soul with the divine (samadhi). A balanced asana practice also depends on ethical behavior (yama) and self-discipline (niyama).

In Astanga Vinyasa Yoga, the first of the six sequences of postures in total is known as the Primary series, or yoga *chikitsa* (therapy), and is designed to cleanse and purify the internal organs of the body through preventing an accumulation of waste matter. Each series, like asanas, has specific benefits, such as forward-bending postures, which are focused on in the Primary series, and which are helpful in toning and relieving constipation. The Intermediate series, for example, focuses on back-bending postures. The remaining four series are extremely advanced and seldom taught, particularly here in the West, though there are exceptions and I have known both men and women who have advanced to the third and fourth series.

The Astanga Vinyasa Yoga system places equal emphasis on strength, flexibility, and stamina, and is thus one of the more challenging asana schools. This is not a practice tailored for the beginner for a number of reasons. For one, you need to memorize the series by studying under someone who is him- or herself an advanced practitioner so that he or she can assist you in aligning your body into positions you may not be able to reach on your own. Also, this is traditionally a six-day-per-week practice. Saturdays are the only rest days of the week, apart from new moon days. Astanga Vinyasa requires a lot of discipline in order to advance to the next series, but through the discipline of rigorous repetition, you can suddenly find yourself doing things with your body that you never imagined possible.

Today, many yoga centers across America offer "Astanga" classes. Be wary of those who use this name without an explanation of the practice or indication of whether it is a Primary series or not. Every series begins with Suryanama Skara, sun salutations, which creates the flow of vinyasa and ujayyi for the entire practice. If you are interested in pursuing this practice for yourself, it would be a good idea to first speak with the teacher of the class to get a better sense of his knowledge of this practice and where he is in his own prac-

The Eight Limbs of Yoga (astanga)

1. YAMA

Attitudes toward our environment—comprising *ahimsa*, the Hindu ethic of non-violence, restraint from lying, stealing, greed.

2. NIYAMA

Attitudes toward ourselves—comprising cleanliness, serenity, study, devotion, and asceticism.

3. ASANA

Posture practice—positioning of the body while incorporating the breath to achieve a greater awareness in the mind.

4. PRANAYAMA

Breath-control—energizing and balancing of the mind-body through the stilling and flow of breath and prana.

5. PRATYAHARA

Sense-withdrawal—relaxation and internalization of the senses in order to activate the mind.

6. DHARANA

Concentration—focusing and holding of the attention.

7. DHYANA

Meditation—prolonged concentration fills the whole consciousness.

8. SAMADHI

Ultimate state of self-realization—absorbed concentration leads to the "ecstatic" state, the "awakened" state, or liberation.

tice. Generally, one should not teach the Primary series if they have not graduated from the series themselves. There is an extensive Astanga *sangha* (community) in the world today, which can be accessed over the Internet on www.ayri.org, a great resource for finding qualified teachers near you. Typically, classes are led in the Mysore style, which means that an experienced teacher oversees your practice, carefully monitoring your progress along the way.

The following is the invocation that is recited aloud at the beginning of each session or class in unison.

"The Astanga Vinyasa Invocation"

Vande Guruṇāṁ Charānaravinde
Sandrśaita Svātmasukhāva Bodhe
Niśhreyase Jāngalikāyamāne
Saṁsāra Hālāhala Mohaśāntyai

Ābāhu Puruṣākāram
Śaṅkhacakrāsi Dhārinaṁ
Sahasra Śirasam Śvetam Praṇamāmi Patañjalim.
OṀ

I bow to the lotus feet of the guru who awakens insight into pure happiness of pure Being who is the refuge, the jungle physician who eliminates the delusion caused by the poisonous herb of *samsara* (conditioned existence).

I prostrate before the sage Patanjali, who has thousands of radiant, white heads (in his form as the divine serpent, Ananta) and who has, as far as his arms, assumed the form of a man holding a conch shell (divine sound), a wheel (discus of light, representing infinite time) and a sword (discrimination).

Other renowned Astanga Vinyasa Yoga teachers:

1. Eddie Stern, the founder of the Patanjali Yoga Shala in lower Manhattan, New York, and the publisher of Pattabhi Jois's *Yoga Mala*.

2. Chuck Miller is the co-director of Yoga Works in Santa Monica, California. He conducts yoga workshops and seminars internationally along with his life partner, Mati. Chuck has studied with Pattabhi Jois for over twenty years.

3. Richard Freeman is the director of the Yoga Workshop in Boulder, Colorado. A student of yoga since 1968 under the tutelage of Pattabhi Jois in Mysore, India, Richard continues to teach regularly at his own center and in workshops around the world.

The Iyengar Method

Iyengar Yoga is taught and named after another of Krishnamacharya's students, B. K. S. Iyengar, who chose to find the meaning of the sutras through practical study and regular self-practice. Iyengar teaches that all eight aspects of Astanga are also integrated in the practice of asana and pranayama, and that these practices can teach anyone to concentrate on any subject of his choice, thus exercising the mind. Iyengar also reveals how an individual can develop her discriminative faculties, whereby she can better differentiate the essential from the incidental—not only to attain physical poise, but also mental peace, intelligence, clarity, and emotional equanimity. Iyengar teaches that the performance of an asana requires disciplines inflected with yama (ethical behavior) and niyama (self-discipline), and that the body itself should be guided by asana. In Iyengar Yoga, the roles of pranayama, pratyahara, and dharana, while doing the asanas, will lead the practitioner to experience the highest levels of Astanga— antaranga and antaratma sadhanas.

Iyengar Yoga can be practiced by anyone, and

Other schools derivative of the teachings of the Iyengar Method and some reputable teachers affiliated with B. K. S. Iyengar:

1. Patricia Walden is the Director of the Iyengar Yoga Center of greater Boston and leads classes and workshops internationally. She began studying with B. K. S. Iyengar in 1976 and plays an active role in the Iyengar Yoga community. Patricia has a variety of yoga videos available on the market, many of which are frequently advertised in *Yoga Journal* magazine.

2. John Friend is the founder of Anusara Yoga, a system that integrates bhakti or devotional yoga with universal principles of alignment, and is author of *Anusara Yoga Teacher Training Manual* (Anusara Press, 1999). John began practicing asanas in 1973 at the age of thirteen, and went on to apprentice several teachers of different traditions until 1989, when he went to Pune, India, to study with B. K. S. Iyengar. John is also a Siddha Yoga devotee.

3. Rodney Yee is the co-director of the Piedmont Yoga Studio in Oakland, California, where he teaches regular classes and also retreats and workshops around the world. He is featured in over twenty-six yoga videos and has recently co-written his first book, *Yoga, the Poetry of the Body* (Gaiam, 2002).

focuses primarily upon standing asanas. Precision and alignment are emphasized in all postures, and students are encouraged to stay for long durations of time in each posture so as to fully experience it. Props such as belts, ropes, and blocks are used in this practice to allow you to strive for further perfection within each posture. Once you have mastered a level of comfort using the props, you can learn to re-create the posture with the same precision without them. Props also allow you to experience the benefits of the classical postures that you may not be able to attain without their support. Iyengar Yoga does not teach meditation, because dhyana is a state believed impossible to be taught.

Iyengar teaches that, through the practice of yoga, you can become the best that you can be at whatever you apply yourself to. However, a posture practice performed without the total involvement of the mind and intelligence becomes merely exercise, and not an asana. Asanas are reflection in action. The subtle body, the emotions, and the physical body cannot be separated. Like Astanga Vinyasa Yoga, Iyengar Yoga is not meant for the casual practitioner (not to be confused with "beginner"). They are both incredibly demanding practices that will require a serious level of involvement, both physically and emotionally, during their practices. Students are expected to perform to their maximum capability, and teachers should constantly raise the standards so that there is always room for improvement and progress.

"In each pose there should be repose."
—B. K. S. IYENGAR

Iyengar Yoga is particularly good for beginners because of the emphasis on proper alignment and the use of props. Sun salutations are used in the Iyengar practice, but not always at the start of class. Each class may begin slightly differently, which helps to refrain from conditioning. Once you understand the postures physiologically, from the bones outward, you can increase your pace without much risk. However, holding poses in even the most basic asanas can often feel more difficult than vinyasa. There are many branches of Iyengar Institutes around the world, which can be located through the Internet.

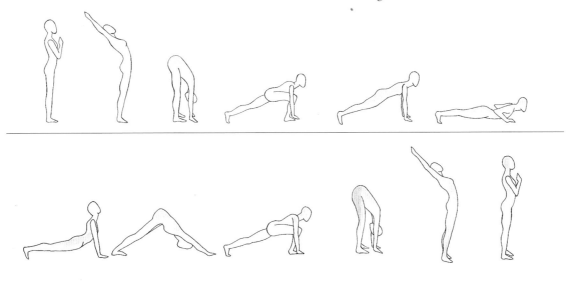

Surynamaskara

Perhaps one of the most balanced cycles of all asana series is *Surynamaskara*, or "sun salutation," as it is commonly known. The sun salutation is an ancient ritual in which the yogi greets the sun. The sun welcomes the day and warms the body, in addition to being a great energy source. An essential routine in Hatha Yoga, particularly Astanga, the sun salutation combines asanas and pranayama, establishing the connection of movement and breath, and mind, body, and spirit. Though it can be a complete exercise in and of itself, it is a wonderful way to begin a yoga practice. The most important aspect to the sun salutation, aside from proper alignment, is the focus and maintenance of a steady synchronized rhythm of the breath and the posture flow. The benefits of the sun salutation are as broad as the range of postures that it incorporates—it tones the digestive and nervous systems, massages the inner organs, stretches the stomach and spine, opens the lungs and oxygenizes the blood, and helps eliminate toxins through the skin, lungs, intestines, and kidneys. Surynamaskara helps increase the body's natural immunity. For the newcomer, the sun salutation is a great way to begin and develop a practice.

The sequence postures are as follows: *samasthiti, uttanasana, chaturanga dandasana, urdhva mukha svanasana, adho mukha svanasana, uttanasana,* and *samasthiti*. Again, as with all yoga, it is advisable to begin a practice with a guru master or experienced teacher so that you will learn proper alignment and breathing.

Kundalini Yoga

Kundalini Yoga, or "The Yoga of Awareness," is taught by Yogi Bhajan, Ph.D., a *Mahan* or master of White Tantric. Until 1969, Kundalini Yoga was kept very secret and only passed down selectively and verbally from a master to the chosen disciple. Bhajan made it more accessible after recognizing that this form of yoga could be particularly helpful to recovering addicts, because he believed it to be the fastest way to heal their bodies and minds and give them the spiritual awakening they were seeking. Kundalini Yoga is an invigorating practice that can stimulate the nervous and immune systems, also improving strength and flexibility, while helping to center your mind and open your spirit.

The word *kundalini* literally means "the curl of the lock of hair of the beloved." It is a metaphor used to describe the flow of energy and consciousness that already exists within each one of us. Kundalini also refers to the serpent energy in the spine, which, once awakened, can lead to a euphoric state.

Kundalini Yoga can be applied to our bodies and minds, but it is aimed at our spirit, which has no boundaries and does not discriminate.

Kundalini Yoga is the practice for what Hindus and Buddhists refer to as "householders"—those who have to cope with the daily challenges and stresses of holding jobs and raising families. Kundalini Yoga, like all yoga, is designed to give you a direct experience of your highest consciousness. It teaches practical methods by which you can discover and achieve a more sacred purpose of your life.

Kundalini Yoga deals specifically, more so than other yoga practices, with prana (life-force energy). Kundalini Yoga is a discovery of the source of the prana within us and the teaching of how to use that energy. It attempts to "harness the mental, physical, and nervous energies of the body and puts them under the domain of the will, which is an instrument of the soul." On a physical level, Kundalini Yoga claims to "balance the glandular system, strengthen the nervous system, and enable the practitioner to harness the energy of the mind and the emotions" so that we can be in charge of ourselves, rather than being so frequently controlled and distracted by our thoughts and feelings.

Kundalini Yoga consists of simple yogic techniques that can be enjoyed by everyone from beginning to advanced levels of yoga. It is believed to be a complete science that includes pranayama (breath), asanas (postures), and sound through mantra chanting and meditation. It is specifically designed to help you experience your highest consciousness through the awakening of your kundalini or shakti energy.

A typical Kundalini Yoga class might begin with some variations of Hatha Yoga asanas and pranayama exercises such as *kapalabhati,* or "breath of fire," until a lot of heat is created in the body and the lungs are expanded.

Another well-known Kundalini Yoga teacher is Gurmukh Kaur Khalsa, the co-founder and director of Golden Bridge Nite Moon Yoga center in Los Angeles, California. A *Sikh* for nearly thirty years, she teaches classes in Kundalini Yoga, meditation, and pre- and post-natal care. Gurmukh also created the popular video series "The Method: Pre- and Post-Natal Yoga" and authored *The Eight Human Talents* (HarperCollins, 1997).

The teacher then slowly unwinds her students toward the climax of the practice, which is ultimately meditation. Meditation here is often accompanied by the sound of a gong while in *savasana,* or corpse pose, which helps bring you deeper into your own subconscious as you rest. More information about Kundalini Yoga can be found through Yogi Bhajan's own 3HO (Healthy, Happy, Holy Organization) Foundation's website, www.yogainfo@3HO.org.

Bikram Yoga

Another popular form of yoga today is Bikram Yoga. Bikram Yoga is named after and taught by Bikram Choudhury at the Bikram College of India in Los Angeles, which he founded in 1974. Bikram studied with his guru, Bishnu Charan Ghosh, brother of the famous Paramahamsa Yogananda (Paramahamsa Yogananda founded the Self-realization Fellowship and also wrote *Autobiography of a Yogi*). Bikram Yoga is unique in that the studios in which the asanas are practiced are heated to over 100 degrees Fahrenheit with 70 percent humidity. The heat is said to be necessary for his twenty-six-posture series, scientifically designed to enhance the mind and body by warming and stretching muscles, ligaments, and tendons. "These twenty-six poses are meant to systematically move fresh, oxygenated blood to each organ and fiber of your body, and to restore all systems to healthy working order," Bikram states in his book, *Beginning Yoga Class*. He believes that in yoga, "there is no standard of comparison except yourself. Perfect is the best you can do

that day." Of the twenty-six poses, two are pranayama exercises, one at the beginning of the class and the other at the very end of class.

Bikram Yoga is steadily gaining popularity, due in large part to the lack of spiritual influence in the classes. It is also practiced in front of mirrors, so the emphasis is unavoidably on the physical. Though some people simply cannot endure the intense heat, others love the fact that you perspire so much, which can leave you feeling deeply cleansed. Today, there are over 100 Bikram Yoga centers and 600 certified teachers around the United States. The twenty-six poses were selected with beginners in mind, but students should use caution when practicing Bikram Yoga because the heat may allow you to be more flexible at that moment than you may have ever been, which could result in subsequent pain and body aches following your practice. Those with low blood pressure or multiple sclerosis should consult a doctor before attempting this yoga.

YOGA INSTITUTIONS

In addition to the yoga schools already mentioned, which are taught by those individuals who have received training and certification from a direct source of knowledge within that tradition, there are also several well-known yoga institutions around the world that provide knowledge, instruction, and resources for the yogi.

Siddha Yoga

A *Siddha* is a perfected yogi, one who has attained the state of unity-consciousness, or enlightenment. The Siddha lineage is an unbroken chain of supreme masters that originates with Lord Shiva. In modern times, the lineage was passed down from Bhagawan Muktananda to Swami Chidvilasananda (also called Gurumayi). Muktananda received the power of the Siddha lineage from his guru, Bhagawan Nityananda, in 1961. The first ashram devoted to the teachings of Siddha Yoga was established in Ganeshpuri, India, but after Muktananda toured America in 1970, others were soon opened in Oakland, California, and South Fallsburg, New York, where Baba Muktananda founded the main SYDA Foundation. In 1982, Baba took *mahasamadhi,* the scriptural term for the passing of a saint, and bequeathed his knowledge and power of the entire lineage on to Gurumayi, the first woman to hold this highly-regarded seat.

Today, Gurumayi travels the world over, chanting with thousands over satellite telecasts or "Global Intensives," which are forums to initiate devotees through *Shaktipat*—"the descent of grace"—or the transmission of spiritual power or shakti from the guru to the disciple or through a spiritual awakening by grace. Workshops and courses are offered throughout the year, and are taught by qualified Siddha Yoga swamis (monks) in a university campus–like setting. To learn more about Siddha Yoga, you can do so by visiting their website at www.siddhayoga.org.

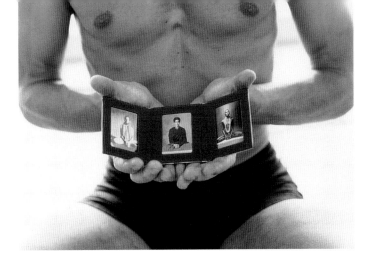

SIDDHA YOGA LINEAGE—MUKTANANDA, GURUMAYI, AND NITYANANDA

Kripalu Yoga

Kripalu Yoga refers to itself as the "yoga of consciousness," or the "willful practice." This school of yoga was developed by the founder of the Kripalu Center of Health and Healing, Amrit Desai, in Lenox, Massachusetts, in 1966. Kripalu Yoga is also based on Hatha Yoga postures, with an emphasis on listening to your own body for feedback throughout the postures. The goal of this yoga school is psychological, as well as physical. Like some of the other schools we have already reviewed, Kripalu Yoga aims to make its principles both applicable and practical to daily life.

The Kripalu philosophy of teaching has evolved from the guru-disciple tradition to a paradigm of self-sourcing and self-empowerment by the student. This paradigm is designed to provide the tools to help individuals seek their inner wisdom and find support for the ongoing process of growth and spiritual development. The Kripalu Center for Yoga and Health was named after Desai's own guru, Swami Kripalvananda, who was a renowned master of Kundalini Yoga. In addition to yoga, Kripalu offers courses that range from Shiatsu training to Qigong and Tai Chi, through their Healing Arts program. Yogi Desai resigned as spiritual director in 1994. For more information, visit www.kripalu.org.

Integral Yoga

Integral Yoga is a system for the harmonious development of every aspect of the individual. Integral Yoga, as taught by Sri Swami Satchidananda, is a synthesis of methods that develops all sides of the spiritual aspirant. The different branches that together create Integral Yoga are the following six practices: Raja Yoga; Japa Yoga, the repetition of a mantra; Hatha Yoga, *kriyas* or cleansing practices to purify and strengthen the body and mind; Karma Yoga; Bhakti Yoga; and Jnana Yoga. For more information, please visit www.integralyogaofnewyork.org.

Ardha baddha padmottanasana

Ardha means "half," *baddha* means "bound," *padma* means "lotus," and *uttana* is "a stretch." This posture, an intermediate step in the ardha baddha padmot-tanasana, combines the benefits of acquiring balance and standing firmly exercised in tadasana (mountain pose) with stretching the leg muscles.

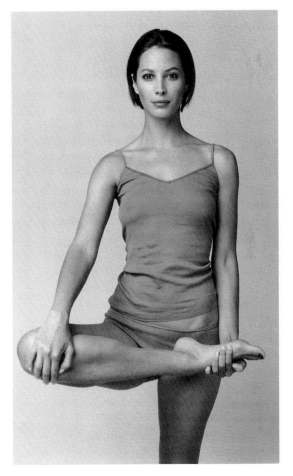

Prasarita Padottanasana I, II

Prasarita means "expanded" or "spread apart." *Pada* means "foot" or "leg." In this posture, the legs are stretched far apart. In the advanced stages of this asana, the hands can be placed on the waist, instead of the floor, or folded at the back as if in prayer, or stretched out in front of the practitioner with her fingers interlocked (these hand gestures help open up other areas of the trunk, as well). With the feet spread wide apart, toes pointed only slightly inward, and the practitioner bent over, this posture increases blood flow to the brain and lengthens the spine. The hamstring and adductor muscles are also stretched and flexibility is increased. Also, grasping your big toes and drawing your elbows to the sides opens up the collarbone region.

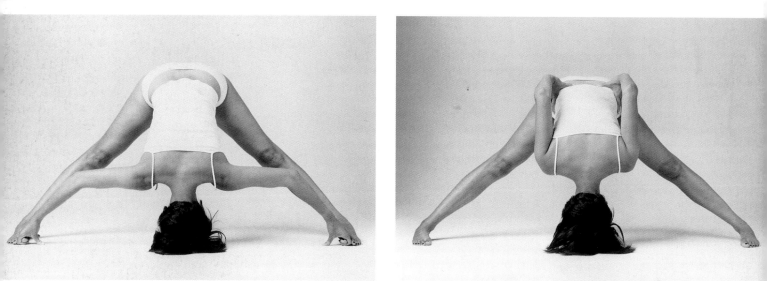

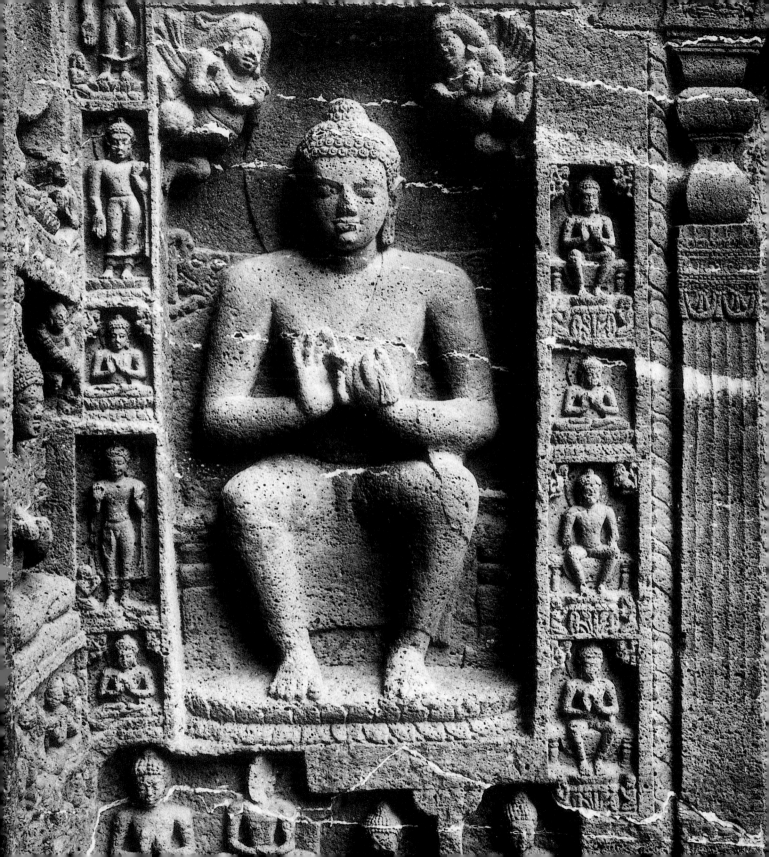

THE PATH

"A good traveler has no fixed plans, and is not intent on arriving."

—LAO-TZU

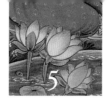

5

The path to enlightenment—and more practically,

the path to mental, physical, and spiritual peace

—begins, like most journeys, with a leap of faith.

Through philosophical enquiry or just a basic surren-

dering of that something we refer to as "ego," we

may take the first steps of learning. Freedom from

the ego is the primary spiritual goal of most Eastern

religions. In Hinduism, every action in the world

results in either a closer binding of the individual

soul (atman) to the world of illusion, or nearer to the detachment thereof. The ultimate spiritual goal for Hindus is to achieve moksha (liberation), the state of spiritual perfection that allows the soul to be released from all worldly ties. The negation of the ego is also the premise for enlightenment in Buddhism. For both of these religions, and particularly in religions such as Judaism, Islam, and Christianity, faith is required in order to discover inherent truth in oneself and in teachings.

While faith is the great universal stepping-stone, it is important for us to realize the complexities and challenges of a spiritual path. In addition to written texts, we often seek the guidance of a companion or skillful teacher to stimulate and encourage us. For Christians, that teacher is Jesus Christ. For Muslims, it is Muhammad. In Hinduism, and in yoga, the path of knowledge (*jnana-marga*) and the path of devotion (*bhakti-marga*) are embarked upon with the guidance of a guru, a personal spiritual guide. Some bhakti, or devotional, traditions pursue the surrendering of the ego under the consideration of a teacher's wisdom that is integral to a student's fulfillment. Being in close proximity to

a guide—a realized being—sheds light onto you, which can ignite your own realization and help you along on your own path.

For Buddhists, and even for many other believers, the Buddha is an exemplar of gurus. In Buddhism, all great teachers, and the personified ideal to which a student aspires, emulate the Buddha and his own personal life. Born Prince Siddhartha, the Buddha escaped his palatial luxury and fled to the outside world, where he was confronted with the decay of old age, the agony of sickness, and the finality of death. He realized that his own life had been based upon illusions, and so he set out to discover the deeper meanings in human existence. He spent many years "subjugating his body to enable his soul to transcend the physical world. Yet the path of self-mortification did not lead to the true wisdom he desired" (Jane Hope, *The Secret Language of the Soul*, p. 28). He eventually came to rest under the Bodhi Tree, determined to stay and meditate until he reached true understanding.

Reflecting upon the wheel of life, or "Samsara" —the notion of cyclical time and rebirth —Siddhartha came to realize that present experiences were caused by past actions in a process called karma. During the passing of night, he recognized that false adherence to the ego resulted in an illusory sense of self, blocking a person's ability to perceive his or her true nature. Upon this realization, Siddhartha touched the earth in a symbolic spiritual release from that illusory and endless cycle of rebirth. At that moment he became Buddha, "the awakened one," and the insights that he gained throughout that night under the tree became the essence of his teachings on the Four Noble Truths, or *aryasatya*, which is at the core of the Buddhist dharma, or teachings. The Truths explain the ubiquity of *dukkha*, inherent in the human condition, a word implying transience, impermanence, imperfection, and suffering.

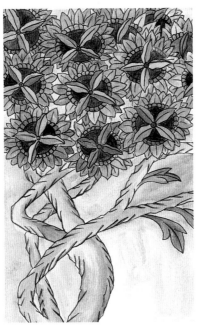

According to the Four Noble Truths, one can escape dukkha by following the Eightfold Path, thus transcending egotism and achieving enlightenment. The Eightfold Path is one of ethical behavior, meditation, and skillful action, and is divided into three "trainings," which are all dependent on one another, according to understanding, behavior, and concentration. This path, which is essentially the Four Noble Truths, reflects the Buddha's specific instructions on how to purify one's heart and mind by living an enlightened life. It is about living in a spiritual way, day to day, through everything we do. Through this path, also called "the Middle Way," we may experience the liberation and insight that the Buddha exemplified.

Buddhism teaches this Middle Way as the way between two extremes of radical asceticism and radical hedonism. Buddhism is a practical religion, with the Buddha as a model for a human being who achieved the goal of nirvana, a state of bliss here on earth. The symbol of his path is a pair of footprints, which represents a sturdy foundation grounded in humility and also impermanence. The footprints are proof that Buddha was here, but now that his physical body is gone, his teachings remain as the guide for others to follow. Buddha walked this same earth and attained nirvana, so we can, too, if we choose to follow the path he created. The feet of anyone perceived to have wisdom or knowledge of the truth are revered by others who bow to touch their feet. The feet represent the path to the truth or to knowledge.

As in many Eastern religions, the emphasis on an enlightened being is not grounded as much in historical accurateness as in symbolic or mythological significances. Before the time when Buddhism became established, there were two possible destinies one could have: that of a renunciate, or of a householder. A renunciate, or *sadhu,* was one who relinquished his worldly responsibilities to follow a spiritual path in solitude, surviving upon the kindness of strangers. A householder maintained his familial and professional obligations while simultaneously pursuing a spiritual life. Many householders in the East choose to renounce their obligations toward the end of their lives.

When traveling in India, I always look into the faces of these sadhus, who are often barefoot and dressed in tattered orange robes, walking on the side of the roads carrying their small tins for food and water at their sides. I try to imagine what situations these enlightened beings have left behind; how often they think of their earlier lives and families. The Catholic Saint Francis of Assisi, whom the Franciscan order of that church is named after, also renounced his secure standing in a prosperous family on his personal path of enlightenment. But, of course, it is not necessary to become a renunciate to embark on a spiritual quest. Nor is it necessary to become a Buddhist to do so, as you will find.

To clarify, the eight limbs of yoga are the predecessors to the Buddhist Four Noble Truths and Eightfold Path, which prescribe a similar path to enlightenment (to Hindus, the Buddha is accepted as an incarnation of the Hindu deity Vishnu, thus creating the moment from which Buddhism grew). Again, this path, the practice of yoga, seems to have first been suggested in the famous epic poem the Mahabharata, specifically in the Bhagavad Gita. There are many different ways to pursue clarity through yoga. The four main paths of

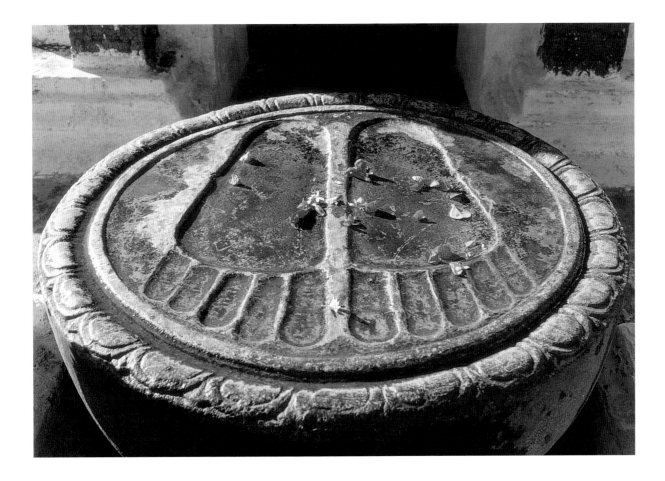

yoga are: Karma Yoga, Bhakti Yoga, Jnana Yoga, and Raja Yoga, which were briefly mentioned earlier on. Each is suited to a different temperament or approach to life, in order to appeal to everyone. However, like the Four Noble Truths, all paths lead to the same goal: union with atman (individual self), Brahman (universal or supreme self), or God.

Karma Yoga is the yoga of action. It is generally the path chosen by those with an outgoing or extrovert nature. It purifies the heart by teaching you to act selflessly, without thought of gain or reward. By detaching yourself from the fruits of your actions and offering them up to God, you learn to sublimate the ego. Through Karma Yoga, we involve ourselves in

The Eightfold Path

Clear understanding of the Four Noble Truths and the intention to act accordingly

STEP 1. RIGHT VIEW

The realization that the true nature of the world involves good and bad, and the understanding that there is no self.

STEP 2. RIGHT RESOLVE

The realization that the quality of an act is determined by its intention, therefore one must renounce unhealthy and temporal desires, ill intentions, and harm against oneself and others.

ETHICS TRAINING, OR VIRTUE:

The disciplining of one's intentions and behavior

STEP 3. RIGHT SPEECH

Restraint from lying, harsh language, and idle talk.

STEP 4. RIGHT ACTION

Abstaining from killing, stealing, and illicit sexual intercourse.

STEP 5. RIGHT LIVELIHOOD

Abstention from practices that harm living creatures, such as deceit, fraud, usury, soldiering, hunting, and the selling of weapons, liquor, slaves, or livestock.

MEDITATION TRAINING, OR CONCENTRATION:

Free from remorse, the cultivation of mindfulness leads to right concentration, consisting of the dhyanas

STEP 6. RIGHT EFFORT

Overcoming harmful and malevolent thoughts and preserving, cultivating, and nurturing wholesome mental states.

STEP 7. RIGHT MINDFULNESS

The focusing on one's body, feelings, mind-states, and thoughts as part of the process of cultivating awareness; the mindful observation of unconscious activities like breathing and movement through various practices such as Theravada.

STEP 8. RIGHT CONCENTRATION

The practice of various techniques, particularly the four dhyanas, to transcend consciousness.

life through our actions, but we expect nothing and are not affected as a consequence by the results of those actions. As in Astanga, yama, niyama, asana, and pranayama are essential components of Karma Yoga because they keep the body and mind healthy for performing acts of devotion.

Bhakti Yoga is the path of devotion or divine love. This path appeals particularly to those of an emotional nature. The Bhakti yogi is motivated especially by the power of love, and sees God as the embodiment of love. Through prayer, worship, and ritual, the practitioner surrenders herself and all actions to God, transferring or channeling her emotions into unconditional love. Chanting or singing the praises or names of God is a substantial part of Bhakti Yoga, in which all that one does and sees is divinely devotional.

Jnana Yoga is the path of knowledge or wisdom. This is the most difficult path, and requires tremendous strength of will and intellect. Taking the philosophy of Vedanta, the Jnana yogi uses her mind to inquire into its own nature. Jnana Yoga leads the devotee to experience unity with God directly by removing the obstacles and dissolving the veils of ignorance. Jnana Yoga assumes that all knowledge lies within us, and through this practice we will discover it. Dhyana provides the way to this discovery, and both dhyana and samadhi help merge the body, mind, and intelligence in the ocean of the Self.

Raja Yoga is the science of physical and mental control. Raja means "king." This path is often called the "royal road" because it includes all eight limbs (astanga) of yoga, and offers a comprehensive method for controlling the waves of thought by turning our mental and physical energy into spiritual energy. These eight limbs also lead to absolute mental control. The main practice of Raja Yoga is meditation, but it also includes other methods to help one to control body, energy, and senses, and to conquer the mind, connecting with the king within.

There are numerous other paths of yoga, including two of the more common paths known as Mantra Yoga and Hatha Yoga, which we explored in depth in the previous chapter.

As you can perhaps guess, Hatha Yoga is probably the most widely-practiced path in the West, as it is the type of yoga that incorporates the physical postures (asanas). The Hatha yogi also uses pranayama (relaxation), which will be further explored, as well as yamas, niyamas, mudras, and *bandhas* to gain control of the physical body and the subtle life-force energy (prana). Hatha Yoga understands that when body and pranic energy are under control, meditation comes easily and awakening ensues. Because Hatha Yoga is the physical practice that most of us are familiar with (when we talk about yoga "poses" we are talking about Hatha Yoga), and since it is that path that we may first choose to explore at our nearest yoga center, I have focused much of the information in this book on the various practices within and applications of this most accessible yogic path.

Most of all, remember that no matter what path you choose, yoga is about you and about being alive. It is a journey about discovering who you are and learning to listen to what your body is telling you.

Parivrtta Parsvakonasana

(revolved side angle pose)

Like utthita parsvakonasana, this asana is a lateral angle posture. The difference in the two postures is that parivrtta parsvakonasana is a revolving pose (*parivrtta*

means "revolved" or "turned around"). This posture is a more intensified variation on the extended lateral pose, and thus has a greater effect. The hamstrings are not stretched as fully as in the revolved triangle pose; for example, the abdominal organs are more contracted and digestion is more greatly aided. This posture increases circulation around those organs, as well as the spinal column, returning vitality to the area.

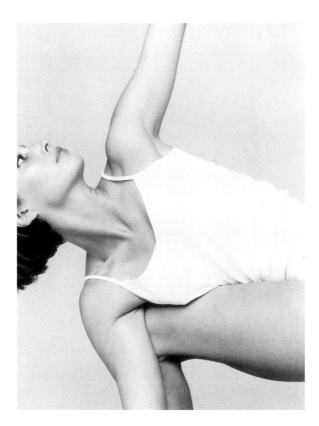

KARMA YOGA

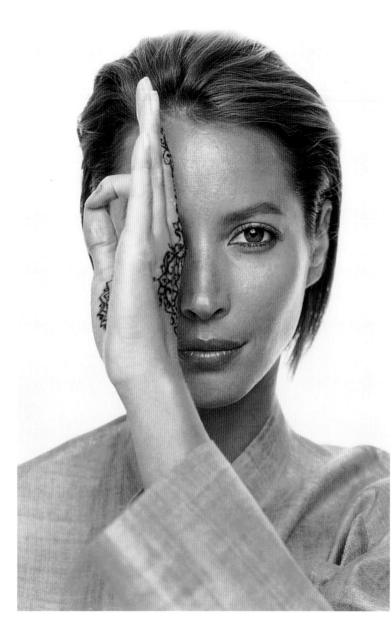

"Each relationship is energy. The concept of sangha, for instance, means a group of people working together as brothers and sisters, working together as spiritual friends to one another. . . . In order to be spiritual friends, you have to be open to each other. . . . Being open is not being dependent on others, which blocks their openness. In other words, the sangha does not create a situation of claustrophobia for each person in it. If somebody falls, you still stand independently; because you are not leaning on the other person, you don't fall. When one person falls, it doesn't create a chain reaction of other people falling as well. So independence is equally important as being together, acting as inspiration to one another."
—CHOGYAM TRUNGPA RINPOCHE

"All of life is relationship, and it is how we relate to people, to things, to ideas, and to our past actions that defines who we are."
—JOHN MCAFEE

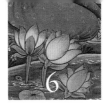

6

Discovering the delicate balance between creating

meaningful and sustaining relationships while main-

taining your independence can be one of life's great-

est challenges. It is somewhat like striving toward the

balance of achieving inner peace as well as outer

peace. In fact, it may be that very same challenge, or

at least a representation of the same principles at

work, which at times may seem impossible. Learning

to experience the world with equanimity in all

respects is part of the goal of yoga. Understanding the self better should, in turn, help us to better understand "the other," just as traveling abroad helps us to better understand our own communities, and also teaches us to appreciate all that we are, no matter where we go.

Oftentimes, focusing too much on one aspect of life makes another appear more difficult. In his book *Into the Heart of Truth: The Spirit of Relational Yoga*, John McAfee says that "all of our relationships, from the most casual to the most lasting, are based on either pleasure or fear . . . our relationships bring exploitation, because they are instruments of gratification. This self-centered basis of relationship is the cause of our loneliness and isolation. But true relationship is based on communion, and there can be no communion where there is exploitation . . . our relationships divide instead of join."

The fear of the unknown both outside and inside of ourselves can keep us from experiencing the fullness of who we truly are, as well as our innate kinship to those around us. This can perpetuate feelings of separation from the Self. More fear may then arise from these feelings of separateness, which can only lead to an even more isolated existence, and more fear, than what we may already perceive. These feelings of separateness can only dissolve through a spiritual union, be that with God or another. We can learn much about ourselves through our various relationships with others. Ralph Waldo Emerson once wrote that every soul is a celestial Venus to every other soul.

I have always loved the expression from the Bible that says, "Do unto others as you would have them do unto you." How great a tool we could be for our own comprehension of the Self, if only we could learn to treat others the way that we want to be treated. It is so simple, yet somehow seems difficult to put into practice with any consistency. In relationships, I sometimes wonder if we consciously choose to treat others the way we do *not* wish to be treated, so that we can establish some sense of control and self-protection in the event that a relationship does not work out the way we would like it to. This is where we project our insecurities onto another. The world is a mirror that mimics the reality that we often create in our own minds. What we see around us is the objectification of our own subjective thoughts and beliefs. Most of us have not been taught that how we see things is our own choice. The mirror of the world has no objective reality of its own. Instead, it reflects our own subconscious reality.

The World Is As You See It

We hear the word *karma* thrown around pretty loosely these days. Karma is a law of cause and effect. Originally, in Vedic times, karma referred to the ritual of sacrifice. People would sacrifice something they valued tremendously to nature at first, then to their deity, in order to show thanks to the heavens and also with the hopes of receiving some goodness and prosperity back in return. For them, goodness could have been anything from a fruitful harvest to plentiful rains, or even being spared from plagues. Goodness eventually came to represent God-ness, only much later on. The ancient communities of this time and of the Vedic civilization were quick to discover the power of their actions, and realized that the odds were generally more favorable if they made sacrifices.

In time, the rituals themselves gave more support for this consensus, reinforced by numerous positive outcomes that were, at the time, believed to be controlled by the people themselves. This was, understandably, an empowering discovery, and has since evolved into the organization of the world's religions as we know them today. People of different cultures and ethnicity continue to practice various rituals, passed down from generation to generation, often without knowledge of their true meaning, to ensure that future goodness will come their way. Many of these religions are particularly concerned with the hereafter, while others emphasize achieving happiness in the here and now. But, few consider both with equanimity.

Most of us yearn to "belong," and so we often seek companionship in order to simply feel connected. In truth, we already are *connected* in this web of life, so why is it that we often seem to need another being to complete us?

And, once we do find someone to share our lives with, we tend to hurt one another simply by living out our respective lives. Ideally, we should come to see the other as a complement—someone who brings out the very best qualities in ourselves, and someone for whom we can return the favor. Potential ignites potential.

√ True spiritual love requires openness and trust at every stage. This level of openness will allow each person the freedom needed to develop independently, so that ultimately—together—two become whole. Relationships based on a foundation of truth and love will prevail. Cycles will continue when systems are established and set into motion, be they negative or positive, so if we should choose to perpetuate life through a union with another, it is imperative that we take our commitments very seriously.

I have learned that self-reliance is only an achievement if it allows you the time and space to give and experience more. Otherwise, it is an empty destination. On the other hand, dependence can be quite an achievement if there is total equanimity, where an equal exchange of the spirit is shared. Otherwise, it is eventually debilitating for all parties. Realizing this can help put into perspective the many issues that we face when relating to another. Dedicating ourselves to the practice of serving another can be like a sacrifice exchanged for goodness, or an investment with limitless return. This kind of offering, in the form of a relationship, can be our most important contribution of all to the universe.

"Trust thyself: every heart vibrates to that iron string."
—RALPH WALDO EMERSON IN HIS ESSAY ON SELF-RELIANCE

Utthita Parsvakonasana

Parsva means "side" or "flank," and *kona* is "angle." A good lengthening exercise, utthita parsvakonasana not only tones muscles (alongside the abdomen and waist, down through the legs to the ankles and upward along the arm), it helps one develop stamina, strength, flexibility, lightness, and balance. This posture also relieves sciatic and arthritic pains, and helps digestion.

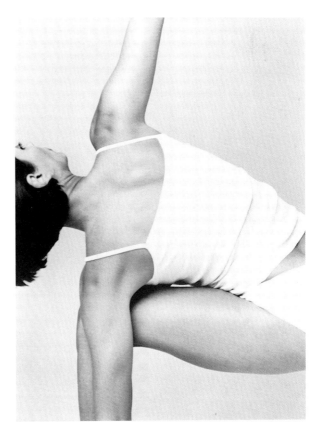

PRANAYAMA (BREATH CONTROL)

"Pranayama is the connecting link between the body and the soul of man,
and the hub in the wheel of yoga."
—B. K. S. IYENGAR

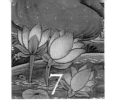

7

Breathing is as essential to yoga as it is to living. In fact, pranayama is integral to every one of the paths of yoga, as breath control is an important factor in the control of the mind as well. *Prana* means "breath," "respiration," "life-force," "vitality," "energy," or "strength," and *ayama* means "stretch," "extension," "expansion," "regulation," "prolongation," "restraint," or "control." Together, they refer to the prolongation of breath and its restraint. More specifically, *prana* refers to the air and life itself.

In almost every yoga class that I have ever been to, the teacher is constantly reminding her students to breathe throughout that practice. It may seem like a funny thing to forget, impossible even, but most of us do in fact tend to hold our breath frequently throughout our daily lives, without even noticing. But, when our breath becomes static, so do we. And it is often only out of sheer necessity that we may be forced to sigh or gasp to get back into the rhythm of the breath.

One of the goals of yoga is the fluidity of mind, body, and spirit. The breath is inherently fluid. We are all accustomed to what is called "voluntary respiration." This is what we are doing throughout most of the day with hardly a thought. And while breathing correctly or with focus may seem quite simple or easy, when you harness your awareness to the breath, you quickly realize that it is more challenging than first anticipated. Pranayama is a complex practice of breathing techniques that involve exercises that have the potential to noticeably affect not only the physical,

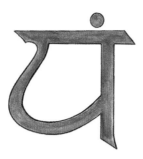

physiological, and neural energies, but also the psychological and cerebral activities, such as memory and creativity. The practice of pranayama develops a steady mind and strengthens your willpower, as well.

Like some of the other facets of yoga, many pranayama exercises may require a qualified teacher and frequent committed practice to fully enjoy their benefits. Iyengar would further argue that it should be taught not just by a teacher, but by a master of the practice as the conscious prolongation of inhalation, or *puraka*; retention, or *kumbhaka*; and exhalation, or *rechaka*. In his extensive text on this subject, *Light on Pranayama*, Iyengar says that "inhalation is the act of receiving the primeval energy in the form of breath, and retention is when the breath is held in order to savor that energy." He also explains, "In exhalation all thoughts are emptied with the breath: Then, while the lungs are empty, one surrenders the individual energy, 'I,' to the primeval energy, the Atma."

"This discipline aims not only at good health, an equilibrium in the physical and vital energies, but also the purification of the whole nervous system in order to make it more capable of responding to the will of the yogi in controlling the sense-urges, and in making the mental powers more subtle and sensitive to the call of the evolutionary urge, the higher divine nature in man."

—B. K. S. IYENGAR, *LIGHT ON PRANAYAMA*

There are a few pranayama exercises that are associated with and often integrated into asanas, as well as various forms of meditation, which I will explain in brief. They are *ujayyi,* or the "victorious breath;" *kapalabhati,* or the "breath of fire"; and *nadi shodhana,* or alternate nostril breathing. While Iyengar believes that pranayama should be taught carefully and apart from asana, Pattabhi Jois's Astanga Vinyasa Yoga has inextricably bound the two together. Iyengar says that the asana must be perfect in order to practice pranayama and, until they are, students should not practice it at all. He also says that when asanas are performed well, pranayama will occur naturally. In Astanga, ujayyi breathing is so greatly emphasized in the practice that a newcomer to an Astanga class may be startled or intimidated by the sound of heavy breathing that inevitably envelops you. However, this community of sound does help to align your own ujayyi breathing, which assists you in the flow of vinyasa (series of postures). When practicing alone, it is like a sort of inner metronome, which serves the body as a measure for the length or duration of a posture.

In Astanga Yoga, ujayyi breathing is also used to enrich prana. Focusing on the ujayyi breath in asana practice causes energy to be channeled throughout the body to support us in difficult postures. If the breath can support you and elevate you in a headstand or balance posture, imagine how useful it can be as a support in difficult emotional situations. In vinyasa, each posture is held for a specific number of breaths, the inhalations and exhalations of which correspond to each movement of a posture, including lifting up into another pose. The breath and gaze, or *drishti,* also have a purpose in each and every asana. For example, on all odd-numbered vinyasa, the gaze should be focused between the eyebrows, and *puraka* (inhalation) should be performed.

On all even-numbered vinyasa, the gaze is on the tip of the nose, and *rechaka* (exhalation) should be performed.

The word and practice of ujayyi refers to an uprising or upward movement of prana. The three characteristics of ujayyi are its very distinct sound, the even flow of breath, and the wave motion that occurs in the diaphragm. Achieving the sound of ujayyi is the most challenging and important characteristic for proper technique of this pranayama. To practice, sit in a comfortable position and draw in the air through both nostrils while holding the back of your throat or glottis partially closed. This partial closure creates a soft snoring sound. The sound should be smooth and continuous throughout the exhalation. It is important to remember that breathing is always done with both nostrils and with a closed mouth. The sound should be heard on both inhalations and exhalations. I have heard it described as though you are breathing through the throat, and not the nostrils. When breathing, the volume of air should remain exactly even, whether exhaling or inhaling.

Once you can breathe evenly with your ujayyi, you can practice it using the wave motion. Think of a seesaw as you begin to fill the chest up, pulling the navel in upon inhalation, then, slowly move the inhalation down until the lower belly is the last part to expand. When exhaling, try to compress the lower belly first by pulling the navel up and back toward the spine and slowly move the exhalation upward until the upper chest is the last to exhale.

Another common pranayama exercise for practicing asanas is kapalabhati breathing. I have found it most useful, in my experience, in postures such as *matsyasana*, fish pose, or *purvottanasana*, the intense east stretch. In Kundalini Yoga, "breath of fire" or kapalabhati is practiced in many asanas. This type of rigorous breathing technique is believed to awaken dormant kundalini shakti energy at the base of the spine, which then spirals upward to the crown of the head, or *sahasrara chakra*, hence the literal translation of the name, "skull shining."

Another purpose of the breath is as a tool that helps keep the mind focused when meditating.

As we will learn in the upcoming chapter on meditation, focusing on the breath is a good exercise, specifically by concentrating on achieving a continuous and steady breath-flow between exhaling and inhaling, just as in the Astanga Vinyasa Yoga asana practice mentioned earlier. Focusing on the breath itself not only has a very calming effect, it is also incredibly rejuvenating for the soul.

Oftentimes, an asana or meditation class begins with the nadi shodhana pranayama exercise, which involves using the right hand in a *mudra* (hand gesture) variation and alternatively closing off the air supply of either nostril and then releasing when the lungs are refilled fully with air, all the while sitting in a comfortable seated posture like the lotus position. This practice clears the mind and awakens the body with increased circulation in preparation for asanas. There are a variety of books available that speak extensively on this subject, but the most highly regarded is Iyengar's *Light on Pranayama*.

Bharadvajasana

This posture is an asymmetrical seated twist, with many revitalizing benefits for the system. Bharadvajasana stretches and strengthens the spine and shoulders, as

well as the hips. Not only does this posture give the practitioner an immediate sense of release, it stimulates the abdominal organs, helps to relieve stress, and alleviates discomfort and stiffness associated with sciatica, arthritis, and backache. Bharadvajasana also aids in aligning the nervous system.

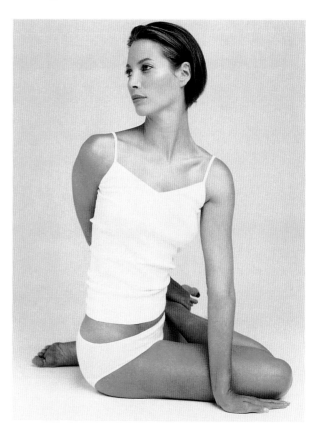

Gomukhasana
(cow-face pose)

In Sanskrit, *Go* means "cow," and *mukha* means "face." With a great stretch of the imagination, this pose is said to resemble the face of a cow. As a sacred animal

in India and as an animal that provides vast nourishment, particularly in the West, with her milk, the cow represents at once a nourishing source of Divine wisdom and a symbol of motherhood. The practitioner of gomukhasana is a receiver of such nourishment. This posture balances the right and left brain hemispheres. And, as we can experience from a meditation practice, deep breathing and the opening of the heart can truly make us feel alive. Gomukhasana opens the shoulders and chest to deepen the breath. Emotionally, feelings of melancholy disappear, and the blood flow to the heart activates the heart chakra and energy is subtly released.

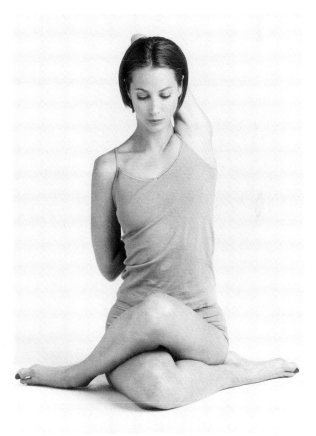

THE BREATH

"As long as there is breath in the body, there is life.
When breath departs, so too does life. Therefore, regulate the breath."
—THE HATHA YOGA PRADIPIKA

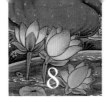

8

For each of us, life begins with our first breath and ends with our last. This act, which many of us do unconsciously, is responsible for sustaining our vital energy, thus keeping us alive. I have come to pay a lot of attention to my breath since losing my father to lung cancer in 1997. He was a serious smoker for more than fifty years of his life. When he was diagnosed, I was not at all surprised, but like him, I knew very little about where the ramifications would lead us when it came time for the inevitable.

As an infant, I suffered from pneumonia, which is probably when I first lost a connection with the essential breath, the unconditioned or voluntary breath we experience as children. One of my grandfathers also died from lung cancer

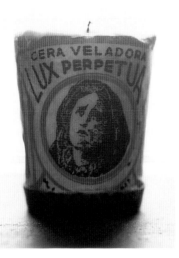

when I was age four, which had a significant effect on me. I can still remember his slight frame sitting up in his bed, the breathing apparatus surrounding him in his small bright hospital room in Southern California, where my mother's Salvadoran family had immigrated in the late 1940s.

Like my father, I, too, began smoking at a very young age. Thirteen, to be precise; long before my lungs were fully developed. A few years later, my dad suffered a heart attack while jogging in the park. He had called his own ambulance from a pay phone. I knew that something bad had happened when my mother came to our school unexpectedly in the middle of the day. I remember seeing my dad, who was six

foot three, in his hospital bed, looking frail for the very first time. It's funny how hospitals shrink the people in them. Like Alice in Wonderland, you feel disproportionate as you're standing over the sickbed or against a wall, trying to keep out of the nurses' way.

It was nearly fifteen years later that my family and I found ourselves in similar circumstances. By this time, following the heart attack, we had moved back home to Northern California from Miami, where we'd been living. My dad had wanted to be closer to his family, while still unable to return to his profession as an airline training captain for Pan American due to his health, which was being carefully monitored by the FAA. He had quit smoking for a while, but eventually gave in to a lifelong addiction because it felt more natural to him than refraining. He carried a small bottle of glycerin tablets wherever he went, and smoked secretly on his own.

The cancer was not quite as sudden as that first warning. The symptoms crept up stealthily. The cough had already become a part of him, but then he started coughing up blood, and feeling general malaise and excruciating back pain. Suddenly, the patriarchy that was my dad's decision-making became a collective process, and all decisions became majority votes in one direction or the other. I was finally in a position where I could show my father, and myself, what I felt for him.

I had already beat my own addiction nearly three years earlier, and had little tolerance for his conscious decision to continue devaluing his life through this habit. Sure, I had struggled as he had, but I finally managed to quit, through *his* encouragement. It was, after all, "mind over matter." Was I lucky, or just sensible? I do not know, but I had set my mind upon something and, finally, I accomplished the goal. But his quitting was also part of my goal. I didn't only want to save myself. When I learned of his suffering, I was able to help in so many ways, but I wanted to do much more. Particularly for my dad.

When I was in my sophomore year at NYU and had just moved into my new home, my father's health took a rapid decline. I turned

twenty-eight that New Year, and went home to find his condition drastically worsened compared to the previous Thanksgiving we'd spent together as a family in New York. He soon opted for exploratory surgery, so we all headed for Minnesota by mid-January to stand by when he went in for the procedure—two families connected by him, our nucleus. All five of his children, two from a first marriage and three of us with our mother, stood around his bed as he slowly recovered from the procedure. When I got there, arriving alone from the East Coast, to meet the rest of the family, he was already fading. "Christy! You're here," he said, then his eyes rolled back into his head as the nurses took him away again and he was wheeled into the operating room.

We learned shortly after the procedure had begun that they'd discovered what we had been told to expect. Cancer was in the lymph nodes, as well as in each lung. Transfusions and transplants are not options for someone who had chosen to smoke all his life, nor at his age (just sixty-three). When he finally woke later that day, he, ignorantly, or hopefully, assumed that whatever it was had been removed successfully. We all stood there, hovering around him, each taking a turn to answer that in fact, no, his lung had not been removed, and yes, he still had "the cancer." The options given were clear, but slim. If he remained there at the Mayo Clinic, they would provide a combination treatment of chemotherapy and radiation. We all opted that he should receive his treatment back home in San Francisco instead, and hoped for the best.

I was able to rearrange some courses to accommodate weekly trips out to San Francisco to surprise him and hold his hand through his first chemo treatments. According to the books, his prognosis was up to five years as in some cases, and we all secretly agreed, optimistically, that this was the term we should adhere to. This was a critical juncture that each of us handled in our own way. I can remember arguing with one of my sisters, who was pregnant at the time, encouraging her to think more positively, because I so truly believed that our states of mind could either uplift or bring down his own state, and thus determine the outcome of his circumstances. Ultimately, the treatment for his cancer triggered other weaknesses in his system and he soon ended up in the cancer ward of a Catholic hospital in San Francisco for his final days.

At the time, hospice was too frightening a concept for us, and his pain too acute to discuss openly amongst ourselves. I had been lucky enough to visit him in that last week, and had experienced his living conditions well enough to know that things had taken a turn for the worse. He was unable to stand on his own, or do much of anything else for himself, so my mom and I together prepared his meals and delivered him to the numerous appointments that would be his last of any kind. You always notice the look on the faces of various caretakers when all hope has been abandoned. A kind nurse taught me a final trick to carry a weakened giant when need be: "Cut open one large garbage bag and have the sick person sit upon it in order to drag him across the hall or room when necessary." That day was the only day I was able to practice this new task, but I will be forever grateful to that kind woman who seemed to know my father's fate. I returned to New York again, promising to be back in a few days' time.

When I returned, he'd been moved from the makeshift room in his house to the San Francisco hospital's cancer ward. I should have noticed right away the significance in the room size. He had been given a large corner room with incredible views of the city. I arrived in from the airport, and he noticed that I was there before heading down for his first and last radiation treatment. He said, "Christy, you're here," before nodding off again. So heavily medicated to control the pain he'd been suffering, he went into a deep coma right after he saw me, and he never recovered from it.

My mother and I were alone together when we had to make the call about whether to resuscitate or not. Making one's own life decisions are heavy enough, but someone else's, with five children and a wife, seemed an impossible task. Everyone was called in just days before Father's Day. Upon arrival, we filled this large room until there was no more space left; the patriarch in the center of it, his children standing vigil over him. Our father was never a particularly religious man, and yet here he was in a Catholic hospital where we asked for his last rites for our peace of mind, and stood

praying over his long, pale body, looking more like a newborn child than a man about to die. He could hardly breathe his last breaths. The nurses periodically brought in oxygen masks and regularly increased his morphine intake, as well, to ease the breathing process. The reality of the value of breathing struck me as I stood witness to his unconscious struggle.

The habit that we'd both found solace in would ultimately prevail and claim his final breaths. I was called into the room for the last time on the morning of June 7, 1997, to witness the final breath of my father. I had stood watching for days, watching the rhythm of his breathing patterns until they at last expired.

A little over a month later, I was visiting my pregnant sister when she went into labor with her second child, Cameron. I drove her to the hospital and acted as her coach until her husband arrived. They had invited me to participate in the birth, since I had missed the birth of her son, who was induced. When we arrived at the hospital, she had already dilated to eight centimeters. She had ordered an epidural, and was adamant that she receive it. In an attempt to relax and distract her, I read from the book *What to Expect When You're Expecting,* simultaneously encouraging her to breathe deeply through the pain of her contractions. A little over an hour later, the top of a little head appeared between my sister's legs. It looked so tiny in the hands of the doctor. When the shoulders were out, they immediately opened up like wings, and then suddenly she was entirely out and separated from my sister's body. Her voice was tiny, too, sounding more like the grunt of a tiger cub than a child. Some fluid had gotten into her lungs, and she needed to have it suctioned out. The doctors took her out, and while Cameron, her father, and my mom were out of the room, I sat with my sister as she cried. Together we had witnessed our father's final breath; and together we witnessed her daughter's first. The miracle of life was not wasted upon us, nor was the miracle of breath.

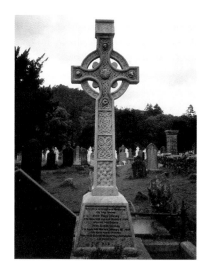

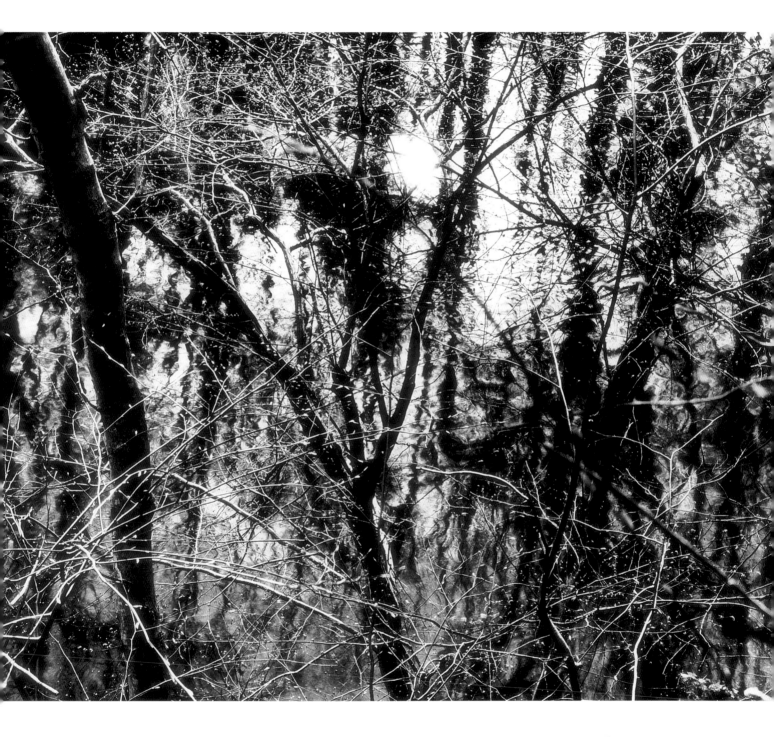

DHYANA (MEDITATION)

"Meditation is a way of clearing away the mental clutter that surrounds the subconscious.
And when our minds are clear, we can see and experience the joy of our own soul."

—GURMUKH

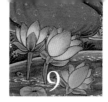

9

The Sufis (Islamic mystics) say, "Knowledge without spiritual practice is like a tree that does not bear fruit." A meditation practice allows the yoga practitioner to live more fully in the present moment with awareness and in peace. The different forms of meditation are as varied and unique as the religious traditions that teach them. Many of us continue to think of meditation as an activity solely involving our minds. Or perhaps we jump immediately to the ideas of chanting and mantra repetition, and imagine robed monks sitting atop a mountain. Meditation is actually a variety of techniques or activities in which we engage our minds and on which we focus our attention.

As we are beginning to see, there are many roads that can lead us to the same place. Therefore, the underlying principles of the posture of meditation are universal in their application—whether you practice Theravadan mindfulness, Christian contemplation, or Hindu mysticism, meditation and its postures are for all seekers. In fact, meditation can and does involve all of these. But, moreover, meditation can be initiated by simply assuming a comfortable seated posture. This gesture, or posture, forms the literal base on which the focused inquiry of meditation ultimately rests and depends. Meditation, or *dhyana,* is the second to last limb of Raja Yoga. In this context, the essence of meditation is explained best in Patanjali's Yoga Sutras: "Yoga consists in the intentional stopping of the spontaneous activity of the mind stuff." Or

"The mind is compared to the surface of a lake ruffled by the wind. And thus the purpose of yoga is to cause the wind to subside and allow the waters to return to stillness. When the wind blows, the waves break and distort the reflections so that they can be seen only as a broken image. When the water is calm, the whole reflection of the sky and clouds appears distinctly and the depths of the water are translucent and clear."

— JANE HOPE, *THE SECRET LANGUAGE OF THE SOUL*

St. Francis of Assisi taught that the aim of meditation (in the tradition of formless meditation in Christian mysticism) is to achieve "a loving, simple, and permanent attentiveness of the mind to divine things." Certain Christian mystics, such as St. John of the Cross, also used meditation as a path to join the presence of God. In order to attain freedom of the soul, it was necessary for the mystics to "liberate themselves from the impediment and fatigue of ideas and thoughts."

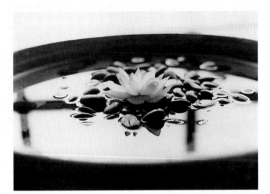

With its roots in the mud, the lotus flower raises itself through the muddy water to reveal its beauty floating clearly on the water's surface. Because of this, this flower symbolizes the rising of the soul from a confusing and selfish place to one of enlightenment. The fully open flower is oftentimes associated with the Buddha (for he sat in the lotus posture as he meditated under the Bodhi tree), but has an iconography ranging from ancient Egypt to Chinese philosophy. The lotus is also believed to signify many opposing concepts: birth and death, male and female, and past, present, and future.

In this light, meditation provides a space in which attention is brought back again and again to the simple yet profound reality of being. Meditation can bring relief from the continuous current of our thoughts and stressful days, offering the soul the space to live fully in the present moment, and to discover a deep delight in the everyday world.

There are as many types of meditation as there are yoga classes to choose from, if not many more. While posture is a very important aspect of meditation, it is not the primary goal. After all, meditation is the stilling of the mind, and it is not always possible to have the perfect environment, or the physical flexibility required in the beginning, to support this posture. To better understand meditation and its invaluable benefits, let's consider one of the greatest "meditators" of all: Siddhartha Gautama, the Buddha, or "the awakened one," meditated continuously for seven days under the Bodhi tree until he finally realized certain truths that he had for so long sought in vain. What he came to realize through meditating became the Four Noble Truths and, through his teachings of them, several different types of meditation have developed. Today, the tradition of meditation has evolved and diverged into a diversity of schools and practices.

Within Tibetan Buddhism alone, there are many methods of meditation. For example, there is the reflection on death, mandala meditation (also *yantra* meditation in Hinduism), and *dzogchen*, which literally means "great contemplation." When considering practicing Buddhist meditation, one must reflect on the idea that there is a Buddha, or Buddha nature, in each of us, and that concentration and questioning are fundamental processes. Many people who meditate in the Tibetan Buddhist tradition—and even those who don't—choose a point of focus, both sensory and non-sensory, to heighten awareness and "go deeper."

Though to most of us it may seem morbid, meditating on death can bring about certain clarities and insights about life. Most of us harbor a significant amount of subconscious fear about death, and act out of this fear in our daily lives. By meditating on death, its

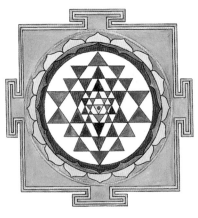

inevitability and yet its uncertainty, it is possible to experience an awakening in this life through realizing just how precious each moment, each mental process, and each breath truly is. A good place to explore this theme is in the *Tibetan Book of the Dead*, an entire text dedicated to the subject of death and dying.

Sometimes, a sensory aid can facilitate the internalization of our awareness for meditation practice. Visualization can be a largely beneficial tool. The mandala is a focusing device, often quite symbolically complex and artistically elaborate, based on the sacred geometry of the cosmos and religious tradition. Often the goal in mandala meditation is to identify oneself with the deity or deities represented in the picture and, furthermore, with the symbolic seed of the universe (the *bindu*). Keep in mind, however, that you don't necessarily have to be a bona fide Tibetan Buddhist to explore these particular traditions of meditation.

Another school of Buddhist meditation is Theravadan meditation, one widely popular method of which is *vipassana* meditation, or "insight" meditation. Vipassana meditation emphasizes awareness and seeing clearly. The practitioner focuses on the impermanent and ever-changing reality of an object or thought. The goal of vipassana is to become so intimate with the idea of impermanence that you naturally come to a place where you no longer depend on the illusion of the permanence of things, the body (also impermanent and constantly changing), or self (as opposed to the Self). Realizing this, as the Buddha taught, we can begin to live our daily lives with mindfulness and gratitude, taking nothing for granted.

A more specific practice related to vipassana is *shamatha-vipashyana* meditation, or "tranquility-insight" meditation. This practice, a basic sitting meditation, along with the practice of *tonglen* and *lojong,* comprises a process by which one is supposed to awaken her heart in order to live a more compassionate life. One of the two very fundamental aspects of this aspirational life is the lojong—a set of teachings belonging to the Mahayana school of Buddhism. Because the Mahayana school rejects full individual liberation and embraces the bodhisattva ideal—that is, a softened

heart and a being dedicated to incorporating social values and helping others on their personal path to enlightenment—these teachings emphasize compassion with and toward all things. Translated, *lojong* means "mind training." Lojong is the practice of working with slogans, simple sayings, to awaken our compassion. Tonglen, the supplement, is a meditation practice designed to help us connect with the full potential of our hearts.

The basic premise of tonglen is taking in and sending out. It is about breathing in suffering, pain, negativity, or anything undesirable, surrendering to it, and connecting with it in the openness of your heart, and breathing out the opposite; ventilating the experience out beyond yourself. While breathing in the negativity and pain, the practitioner focuses on being open and humble enough to bring in what we do not want in our life; the practitioner focuses on the color and texture of it, too (visualizing the breathing in of hot, heavy darkness and breathing out white, cool light).

Another aspect of tonglen is working with a specific object such as the suffering or the anger and the tangibility of such real emotions and situations. Lastly, the practitioner, when breathing out, extends the "sending out" to all other beings because by understanding our own feelings, we can understand that all beings experience similar feelings and suffering. Tonglen is such a wonderful meditation practice, and its beauty is heightened all the more by its adaptable applications —you can use these tools anytime and anywhere. Soon you will be on the path toward compassionate living.

Perhaps you're still wondering what exactly it all means. What is meditation in practical terms, and how can I incorporate meditation into my life? Think of meditation as simply the turning of thoughts inward, the going inside of our selves to probe the questions of deeper levels of consciousness. Sometimes meditation involves repetition, as many yoga practices do begin or end with a simple repetition. In fact, meditation can be as simple as finding a quiet space during the day, closing your eyes, and focusing on a word or a peaceful image. We must come to enjoy the silence because it is good and purposeful. If it is true that the answers are inside of us, we need to quiet the noise of the mind enough to hear our own gentle inner voices. The silence will inform us and guide us to the truth.

Our daily lives are filled with words, but words can either gain or lose their meaning with repetition. It is important to only repeat words that elevate our souls. The rest of it will only deplete our energy source. In silence, we can explore the words that we use all the time and contemplate our actions in inaction. Why did I do that or say this? Observing these processes that we go through is like acting as a witness to ourselves. The deeper we go into the things that we do, the closer we get to the truth. On a more esoteric level, the goal of meditation is liberation from the things that bind us and prevent us from experiencing life as bliss.

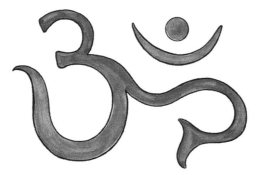

The fact that sound can alter consciousness is another very important aspect of yoga in terms of meditation. Sound is a vibration, and sacred sounds have the potential

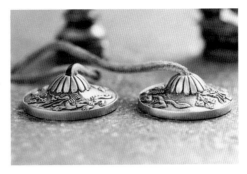

to resonate within us a powerful spiritual flow. One of those sounds is a mantra, the sacred word or cosmic sound invested with the power of God, or God in the form of a sound. A mantra comes from a single sound or a string of sounds that originated during the Vedic period, probably as hymns. But throughout the tradition of yoga, mantras have become known as a meditative tool and consciousness-altering vehicle. Mantras may be repeated mentally and silently (Japa) or spoken aloud. When sung, it is called chanting. When practicing mantra repetition meditation, it is important to reflect on the sound of the word or words and their meanings, and to choose words accordingly. One of the simplest mantras to learn is OM.

OM does not necessarily mean anything. It is merely the sound of the Sanskrit, vowels vocalized, which is inexplicably yet innately familiar. It is the primordial sound in Sanskrit, an ancient Indic language, which is the classical language of India and Sri Lanka. It brings the mind to a calm, primed place, from which a single pointed focus through meditation and asana practices is brought about. Reciting OM alone is also chanting, but when added to other Sanskrit words or sacred names, which resound in vibrations throughout the body, the possibilities become limitless. Chanting Sanskrit is yet another tool to reach enlightenment. Through chanting, the practitioner uses sounds and vibrations to "tune" his or her own consciousness.

OM is a great exercise for beginning any other form of meditation, too. In fact, instead of focusing on the movement of your breath alone, which we discussed in a previous chapter, you could simply work with OM, exploring the full range of the complete sound, A-U-O-M. Some practitioners may also invoke their meditation by ringing a special brass bell, each ring an equivalent of the spoken OM.

In his book *The Teachings of Yogi Bhajan*, Bhajan, a master of Kundalini Yoga, teaches the "Sat Nam" mantra, which is comprised of five primal sounds—*Sa, Ta, Na, Ma*, and a sound that is a common denominator in all four, *Ah*. Meaning "Truth Manifested," Sa Ta Na Ma produces a total vibration proportional to that of all creation. Broken down, *Sa* means totality, *Ta* means life, *Na* refers to death, and *Ma* is resurrection. Bhajan instructs his students to chant this mantra, while alternating touching the thumb to each finger in a mudra, simultaneously to making each sound, in three different ways. First, he suggests chanting out loud, in the "voice of the human being." Then he suggests repeating the mantra as a whisper, in the "voice of the lover." And lastly, Bhajan instructs the student to repeat the mantra in silence, in one's consciousness, in the "voice of God." Chanting in this way, each sound originating in the crown of the head, seated in a meditative posture, it is possible to experience one's "own infinity."

There is also a form of Christian meditation that involves sounds, most commonly as Gregorian chants, which are monadic liturgical chants sung in Latin without musical accompaniment and are named after Saint Gregory I.

I can remember my first chanting experience. I was sitting in a yoga class, and when the teacher instructed us in a call and response style chanting exercise, I opened an eye to look around the room, as if by seeing the mouths moving, I would better understand the instruction and then better manipulate my tongue to pronounce these strange sounds aloud with everyone else. I came to realize, however, that I would first have to look within. Sounds we make begin in the diaphragm and move up and off the tongue. Each time I have chanted, I have gained a better command of the sounds, but it was studying the Sanskrit language at a retreat that really helped me to make the connection between the origins and vowel sounds.

Chanting can be done alone or in a group, but in a group the power of the effect is amplified. Keep in mind that the sounds themselves and the words from which they come are most

Mudras

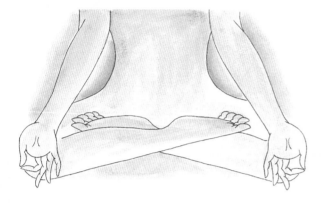

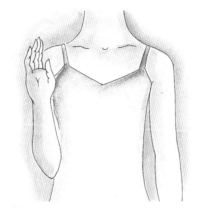

Dana-mudra—the gesture of giving; this gesture is made by extending the right arm over the right knee, with the right palm facing outward.

Abhaya-mudra—the gesture of fearlessness; this gesture, which symbolically dispels fear in others, is made by raising the right hand to the level of the heart and with the palm of the hand turned outward with all of the fingers extending upward.

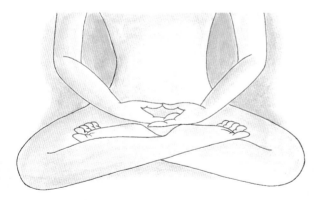

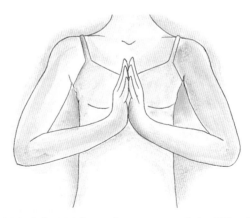

Dhyana-mudra—the meditation gesture; this is done by resting both hands in the lap, palms up, with the right hand on top of the left.

Dharma-chakra-mudra—the gesture of the Wheel of the Law; this gesture is executed differently according to various traditions.

important. It can be scary to chant or speak words that are unfamiliar, so it is important to have some understanding of what is being said. New words and experiences can raise fears, but with understanding and familiarity, the fear will subside. Right intention is crucial in all aspects of yoga. Without understanding the words or language, it will be more difficult to direct your intentions, whatever they may be. Many yoga centers offer Sanskrit lessons so that you can become more comfortable with the pronunciation.

I spent a few days at an intensive retreat a few Christmases ago where the only chant we practiced was OM. There were hundreds of us in one room, and though we were instructed to begin at the same time, eventually everyone had established their own rhythm and the effect resounded at different times. It was like in the children's song "Row, Row, Row Your Boat," where we would overlap each other to the degree that it felt like rushes of waves sweeping over an ocean's surface. This continued for nearly an hour, then the room came to a stilled hush and meditation commenced.

Like OM, chanting usually begins and ends an experience, similar to a clearing of the palate. Even if at first chanting feels uncomfortable, it gets remarkably easier each time. Suddenly you will feel confident, and your voice will boom with the best of them. Once you find which chant you prefer, make it your mantra—something to sing aloud, or to repeat internally, that guides you back on your track. Sound is a powerful healing gift, which most of us have at our disposal.

In addition, OM, like other mantras or chants, is the perfect doorway into your yoga practice. Within the limbs of yoga, meditation is deep reflection or contemplation, which requires *tatiksha* (single pointed focus) that will only improve with practice. Ultimately, samadhi is the true aim of yoga, which must be achieved through meditation. There are two types of samadhi, one of which we can come in and out of, and the other a final or lasting state of bliss when the soul has moved on and the individual soul, or atman, reunites with Brahman the Creator.

For someone who is just beginning, it is good to sit in an easy cross-legged position like *padmasana* on the floor, or to sit in a comfortable chair with your feet directly beneath your knees and a pillow behind your lower back for support. The room can be quiet or, if you prefer, you can play some soft, non-distracting music in the background. Close your eyes and begin to take deep breaths of equal proportion. Count slowly and internally as you inhale and exhale to your full capacity: 1, 2, 3, 4, 5. 1, 2, 3, 4, 5. Breathe in through your nose and extend your belly with each inhale.

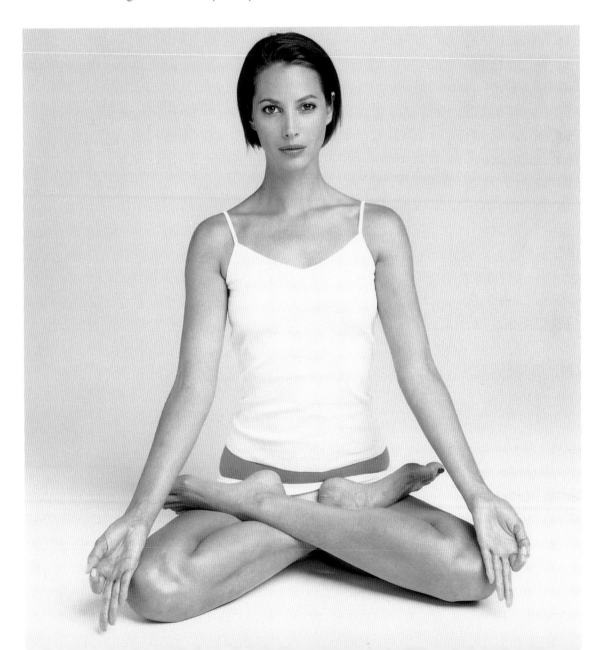

Exhale only through your nostrils. Once you feel you have developed a comfortable rhythm for yourself, stop counting and just follow the breath in and out, imagining a point at which one flows into the other or when the inhale ends and the exhale begins. This is also a form of pranayama.

Witness yourself from outside of yourself sitting there peacefully, and just breathe. While you are trying to stay focused, things will surely come into your mind and begin to distract you. Don't worry when this happens. Be gentle with yourself and your thoughts, and remember that they are just thoughts. Don't get caught up in them. They bring you away from you. Witness them as they come up, and let them go as you exhale and bring your focus back to the breath.

Start with five minutes a day at first, then each week, increase by another five minutes. Soon you will be meditating for a half hour, then an hour; there is no limit. If you find a place in your home where you can make a sacred space for this purpose, go there. Try to make your meditation practice at the same time each day, and eventually you will go into your meditation more easily just by being there. Each time you meditate, it will feel significantly easier to quiet your mind. When you have finally managed to slow your thoughts down, contemplate questions or concerns that you may have in your life. You will surprise yourself with how much you know in this space. You are your own comfort zone.

We often build ourselves up to impossible goals, then sometimes, when we arrive at the goal, we may lose interest or give up, finding ourselves back at square one. If we make attainable goals for ourselves, we will enjoy a more expansive practice. It is important to always challenge ourselves to new heights so that we can experience our full potential, but it is also important not to get too caught up in the goal, so much so that you are unable to enjoy the journey. Eventually, we should arrive at a place where we may choose to surrender the fruits of our goals entirely. And as you have seen, there are many different schools and methods of meditation to explore when and if you so choose, and finding what is comfortable to you can play a pivotal and wonderful role in your daily life.

Prayer

Another related or similar practice to meditation is prayer. Each religion has a ritual of prayer associated with it, and many of these rituals have specific words and practices that accompany them. Like meditation, we often associate prayer with stillness and quiet reflection in a place removed from the distractions of everyday life. In essence, prayer is a communing with the divine (just as yoga can be a "yoking" with the divine). When we pray, we are perhaps searching for inspiration, guidance, or comfort. We may even be asking for assistance of some kind. A famous Christian prayer (many of which were adapt-

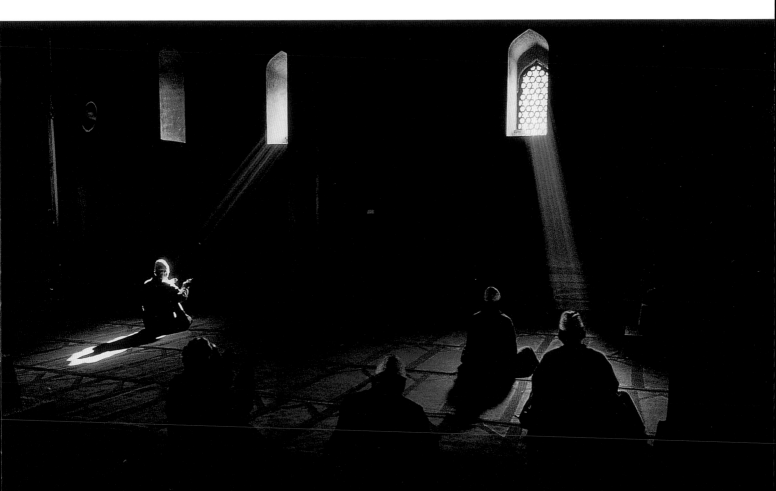

ed from more ancient petitions or pagan gods), St. Patrick's Breastplate, opens with: "I arise today, Through the strength of heaven: Light of Sun, Radiance of Moon, Splendor of Fire, Speed of Lightning, Swiftness of Wind, Depth of Sea, Stability of Earth, Firmness of Rock."

The Jesus Prayer, a supplication of the Eastern Orthodox Church (which also places a strong emphasis on meditative prayer), is used similarly to a mantra. The formula "Lord Jesus Christ, Son of God, have mercy on me, a sinner," was used to effect changes in the consciousness. It was spoken aloud for a specific number of times, and repeated silently throughout the day and night. The chant was eventually taken down from the "head" center of consciousness to the "heart" center, where it was

A favorite prayer of mine is the Lord's Prayer, which I recite every night before going to sleep:

"Our Father who art in Heaven, hallowed be thy name, thy kingdom come, thy will be done, on earth as it is in heaven, give us this day our daily bread, and forgive us our trespasses as we forgive those who trespass against us, and lead us not into temptation, but deliver us from evil, Amen."

believed to live with every heartbeat. Monks used to repeat the prayer while counting knots on a cord. The cord, or some form of a rosary, is still used as a prayer aid in many of the world's religions.

Sikhs, for example, repeat the divine name *nam* while counting the beads on a *simarani* (rosary); Muslims say one of the ninety-nine names of Allah while turning their prayer beads; members of the Pure Land sect of Chinese Buddhists use a rosary while reciting the name of a deified Buddha; Hindus of Kashmir Shaivism (a Hindu sect devoted to Shiva) recite mantras as they pass each bead over thumb and forefinger on their japamalas (beaded bracelets); and Roman Catholics say prayers while counting the beads of their version of a rosary.

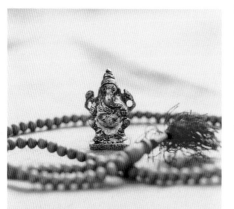

> *"Faith is to believe what you do not see; the reward of this faith is to see what you believe."*
>
> —St. Augustine

While utilizing something such as a rosary to aid us in certain prayers, we often first "submit" ourselves through various bodily attitudes of prayer (bowing, kneeling, prostration). These humble gestures are offerings of reverence, thanks, praise, adoration, contrition, supplication, and so forth. Many religious traditions believe that prayer is at its most powerful when it combines not only reiterated speech, like chanting, but also such physical action. As in bowing or kneeling in Catholicism, for example, the physical postures of yoga are a devotional practice that brings us closer to an understanding of the truth.

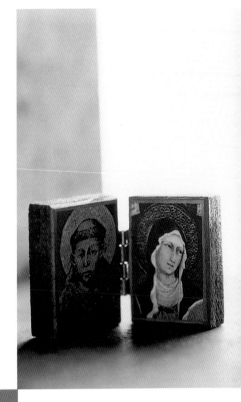

> *"Chanting is a significant and mysterious practice. It is the highest nectar, a tonic that fully nourishes our inner being."*
>
> —Swami Muktananda

"*My country is the world, and my religion is to do good.*"

—Ralph Waldo Emerson

Marichyasana I, II

This asana, named after the sage Marichi (son of the creator Brahma and grandfather of the Sun God, Surya), is excellent for the abdominal region as it causes those organs to contract, thereby increasing circulation. In the more advanced Marichyasana II, the heel at the navel adds extra pressure on the abdomen, thus increasing the effectiveness of the muscle toning and digestive power.

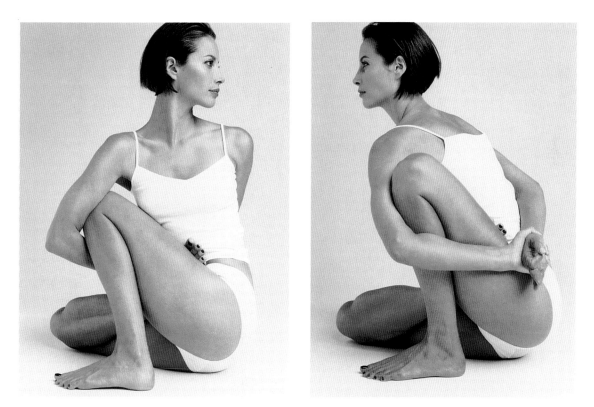

SPIRITUAL INITIATIONS

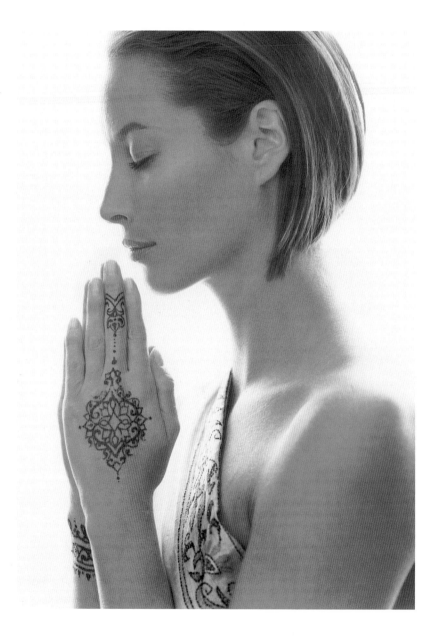

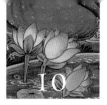

IO

I was baptized a Catholic long before I could under-

stand the meaning of what that was. For most of us,

our religious views are shaped by those of our parents

and communities. My mother was Catholic because

her parents were Catholic, and so on. My father was

not, but allowed my mother to bestow her inherited

beliefs upon our family. In Catholicism, baptism is

the first of the seven holy sacraments, which usually

occurs when a child is still an infant. It is meant to

wash away original sin that the Bible states we mortals have come into the world with. The second is Holy Communion, which occurs when a child is around age seven. This is when we are initiated into receiving the Eucharist, the consecrated bread and wine consumed at the end of mass as a symbolic remembrance of Jesus's life and death. The third is confirmation, at age twelve, which is when a fully initiated individual is admitted to full membership in the church. The other sacraments, all of which I have not experienced, are penance and holy confession, extreme unction, holy orders, and matrimony. The last rites are given in connection with death or at burial. These are the rituals of practicing Catholics.

In my family, my sisters and I were encouraged along this path through our Communions, but we never completed confirmations when we came of age for a variety of reasons, mainly because we had moved to a new community and church, and it was less of a priority with all the newness around us. Because of this, I always felt slightly incomplete within the Catholic church. I never felt that I had understood all of the "etiquette" of the church. I

only knew some of the prayers and recitations in English, not Latin, which led me to feel as though I did not belong. I would sit in church and wait for the parts in the mass that were familiar to me, such as the Eucharist, the Lord's Prayer, and the peace offering. Going to church always felt more like an obligation than a choice. And, though I maintained a connection to that particular faith, for years I would only attend mass on special occasions or on holidays.

Many of us are so tied to the vocabulary used to describe and qualify ourselves to others. These labels, as individuals and as groups, can often cause more feelings of separation than of union, and religions as organized groups have earned a bad rap for contributing further to this imbalance. What does it mean to be Catholic, unless being Catholic is a choice you make for yourself? Today, I am a practicing Catholic. I chose to become one fully in an Easter vigil mass a few years ago.

In the aftermath of my father's death in 1997, and with my recent rediscovery of yoga, I threw myself into my studies and spiritual practice. In addition to focusing my studies on Comparative Religion, I decided to sign up for weekly evening meetings at my church with the RCIA—an adult Catholic initiation program —in order to prepare for a new level of commitment to my faith. I was to be officially welcomed within the Catholic church.

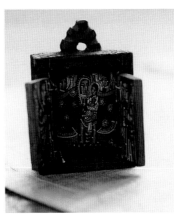

These meetings were comprised of a small group with varied Catholic educations. Our group consisted of a few men and women who were either converting from other Christian religions for approaching marriages or, like myself, had never fully been initiated as adolescents. There was one man who was starting from scratch. His plan was to be baptized, receive Communion, and be confirmed, all in the same night.

At first, I was shocked by how little I knew about the religion I had been linked to for all these years. I learned in school that the first language the Bible was written in was Aramaic, then Greek, then Latin, and finally translated into the other European languages. The word *Catholic* derives from the Greek word "katholikos," which means "universal," which I really liked, so I sought to find those universal truths of the church and the teachings of Jesus Christ. Essentially, the church, like all places of worship, was intended to be the setting for a spiritual community to thrive. We all know that there is strength in numbers and in sharing a collective experience, and this is how I have come to view the church today. This shift in my perception allowed me to realize that it is the experience of unity that brings us closer to God.

On a crisp, sunny Saturday afternoon on the eve of Easter, I scurried off to St. Joseph's for a rehearsal. Up until that day, the church had been devoid of all music and decorative elements for the whole of the Lenten season (a period of penitence for Christians that lasts forty days from Ash Wednesday through Easter). That day, however, it was bustling with activity: Flowers were being arranged, the organ was being tuned, and everything else received a thorough cleaning, all in preparation for the evening's Easter vigil mass.

We all piled in quietly and stood in formation on the dais along with Father Tos, who was going over our cues for the night's ceremony. After rehearsal, we broke for several hours, only to return to the church an hour before mass to change into our white robes. As we lined up in the rectory, we were each given a single unlit candle before the procession began. We then followed the priest out of the rectory, onto Sixth Avenue, and up the steps through the main entrance of the church, pausing momentarily to light our candles from a fire just outside the large glass double doors. Pedestrians threw curious glances at the sight of what probably looked more like a pagan ritual than a Catholic ceremony, mostly because of the Greek revival architecture of the church and the presence of a dozen or so robed adults standing around a single source of fire.

When we entered the seldom-filled darkened church, our fellow parishioners, holding candles of their own, were standing facing us entering at the rear of the church. The flickering flames from all of our candles cast a beautiful glow, like a halo, throughout the room. As we arrived in our procession at the dais and stood in position, the organ music began and the lights came up with a theatrical force, calling our Lord to rise up for Easter.

The mass lasted nearly three hours. We initiates were anointed one by one with the sign of the cross on our foreheads, and then were invited to sit down in the reserved front pews. The final initiate was led from the dais to a side aisle, where he disrobed down to everything but his shorts, which he was wearing beneath his robe. He then walked into the large baptismal font and stood facing us to receive his baptismal rites as we looked on. We were all invited to restate our vows along with this fully grown man as he was doused with blessed holy water. I had never witnessed a more moving ritual than this, and my heart welled up with love at the sight.

After the readings, homily, and Eucharist, everyone was invited back to the rectory for a small feast of home-baked goods and coffee.

It was after midnight. I could sense God's joy in our participation in the celebration of Him, which was emotionally exhilarating. I felt spiritually satiated for the first time that I can recall. The experience allowed me to understand the ritualistic intoxication I would later witness when visiting New York ashrams and Hindu temples throughout my travels to India a few years later.

"For a person who wants to tread the path of yoga, his first effort will have to be to cease to identify himself with the body-life-mind complex completely and to look upon those three elements as tools for transcending the ego, in order to identify his inner being with the pure, unmixed power of consciousness whose very nature is all-peace, harmony and creative joy."

—B. K. S. IYENGAR, *LIGHT ON PRANAYAMA*

Ardha Matsyendrasana
(half spinal twist)

According to Hatha Yoga legend, Matsyendra, a great yogi, was crowned Lord of the Fishes by the god Siva. Lateral movement of the spine, in either direction,

strives to correct lateral curvature of the spine and improve joints in the pelvic region. Rotating the individual vertebrae on each side opens up the areas surrounding ligaments to receive a rich supply of blood. The half spinal twist and spinal twist posture tone and offer relief to spinal nerves, while massaging the muscles of the spine, both deep and superficial. Ardha matsyendrasana helps keep the spine elastic. It also helps massage the abdominal organs, stimulate the pancreas, liver, spleen, kidneys, stomach, and colon. By acting as a tonic for the liver and gastrointestinal tract, this deep twist plays a role in metabolizing and excreting excess hormones, as stated by *Yoga Journal* in October 2001. Regular practice of this posture aids digestion and realigns the vertebral column. Traditionally, it is said to increase the appetite, destroy deadly diseases, and awaken kundalini. It is very important, however, to be patient when practicing this asana, as accuracy in alignment is vital.

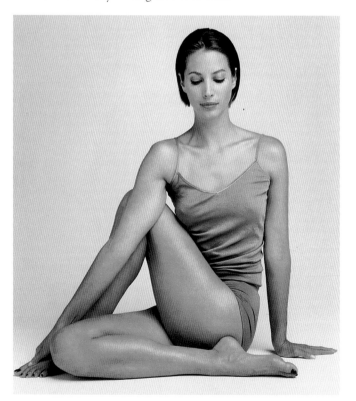

Kukkutasana
(cock pose)

In Sanskrit, *Kukkuta* means "cock" or "fowl." With the legs in padmasana and the hands pushed down through the space between the thigh and the calf, this posture

strengthens the wrists and the abdomen. Though it requires a good sense of balance and concentration (the rooster has a reputation for vigilance), the benefits are valuable. It improves digestive function and stimulates the heart and lungs. Another posture with similar benefits is tolasana (scale pose), which strengthens the wrists, hands, and abdomen, as well.

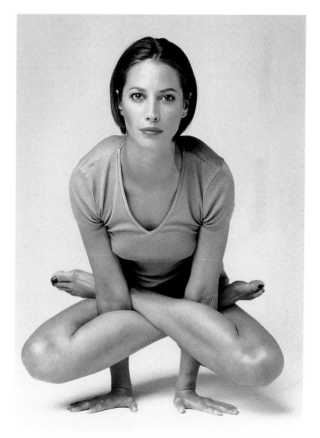

COMPASSION

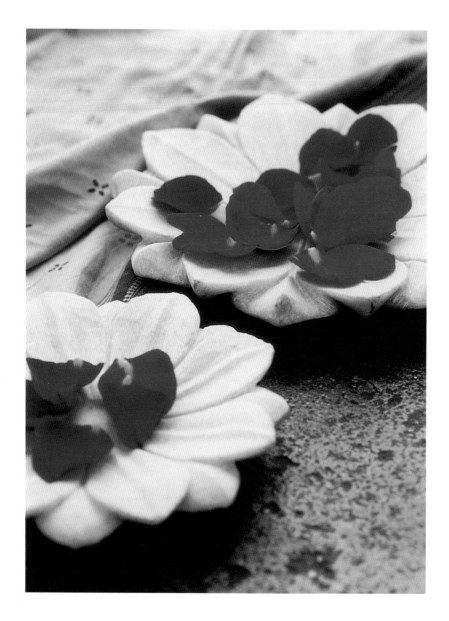

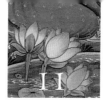

II

As I touched on earlier, many people, including myself, have at one point asked the question, "Can I practice yoga if I am a Christian? A Jew? A Muslim?" Having been raised as a member of a particular religion or sect, it can be difficult to imagine opening up to a practice that has roots in so many other traditions, especially traditions distant from our own. But if we consider yoga as its most basic definition—its true meaning —we realize that yoga in fact transcends religion.

I practice yoga and Catholicism simultaneously, and never feel any disconnect or conflict in doing so. In fact, I feel that my exploration of yoga has deepened my existing faith, because it has opened my mind to such a degree that I see the common sutras or threads in all things. If being a Catholic was originally intended to mean sharing universal values, then it is my duty to broaden my mind as much as I possibly can. Another interesting link is the fact that yoga is always referred to as "a practice," and only when you regularly attend mass are you considered a "practicing" Catholic. To actually "be" something or someone, you must practice it diligently and with regularity. This notion of practice is such an important one, in that it indicates the level of dedication that comes with serious commitment and discipline. Acts of faith done with intention, such as prayer and pilgrimage, become ritualistic, and can bring solace or refuge.

Yoga is proven to predate religion by hundreds of years, so those who may be concerned that they are subscribing to a religion other than their own by practicing yoga need not worry. Hinduism or "Induism" derived from the Vedic age (1500–500 B.C.E.). The Indus Valley civilization, which first inhabited what is now known as India, were a people who recognized the powers of yoga and then applied them to their beliefs to achieve *Brahmavidya* (knowledge of Brahman the Creator). The Buddhists followed suit, but adapted the practices to their own specific needs. Buddha himself reached an enlightened state only after mastering each of the eight limbs of yoga.

One's spirituality is a personal right, so we can worship privately at any time, but historically, worshiping in a group has been an integral part of religion. Temples, churches, and mosques were built with the intention to elevate the spirit through the unity of many. When we come together to worship, the act becomes an exalted experience, just as it does when we come together in tragedy or for a music concert.

As we now know, the goal of yoga is to achieve union with the Absolute, also known as Brahman or Atman, the true Self. To achieve this union is to realize your own oneness with something higher than yourself. One of the beautiful facets of yoga is its openness and versatility, allowing practitioners to focus on the physical, psychological, or spiritual, or a combination of all three. Of course, since they each inform the other, they are most potent when practiced together.

Though we may be constantly aware of our need to fulfill the basic aim of yoga by forming that union with something higher—in order to journey to enlightenment—we must remember to achieve that union within ourselves, as well. We mustn't ever forget that we are part of a far greater web of life than we may know. Through this recognition and path to practice, we may then hope to experience ultimate peace and everlasting joy. Regardless of the path

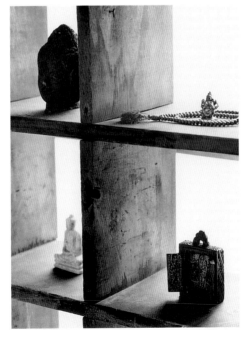

you choose to practice—whether it is through one of the eight limbs of yoga, chanting, simple meditation, practicing asanas, or a combination thereof—our objective is to practice with "mindfulness." Before we *become*, we must *feel*. And once we *feel*, we must learn to *express*.

In Buddhism, one tries to practice mindfulness in each moment. In Christianity, mindfulness can be compared to the Holy Spirit, for both are agents of healing. According to the peaceful Zen Buddhist monk Thich Nhat Hanh, if you have mindfulness, you have love and understanding, you see more deeply, and you can heal the wounds of your own mind. For when you touch deep understanding and love, you are healed.

Bhujapidasana

Balancing on the hands with the legs wrapped around the upper arms and the feet crossed in front of the torso takes a good deal of focus and flexibility. *Bhuja* means "arm" or "shoulder," and *pida* means "pressure." In this posture, it helps to squeeze the arms with the legs toward the midline, which will bring some lightness into the asana. Bhujapidasana cultivates strength in the hands and wrists, as well as in the abdominal muscles. It also helps tone the arms.

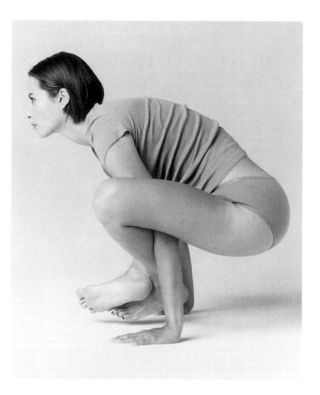

Tolasana
(scale pose)

Tola means "scale." Much like kukkutasana, this posture strengthens the hands, wrists, and abdominal walls.

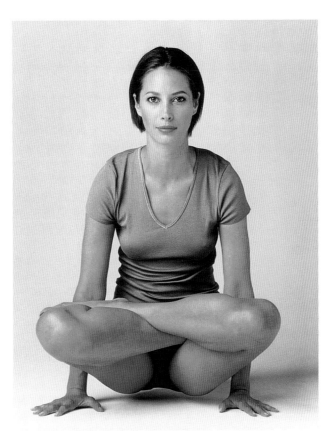

FAITH

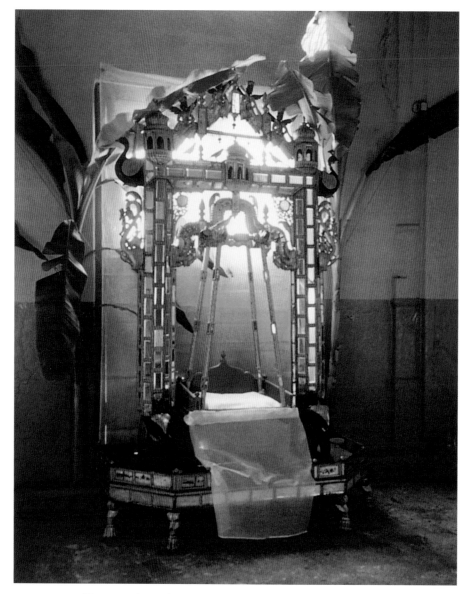

HINDOLA (SWING) SET UP FOR THE SPRING FESTIVAL OF HOLI

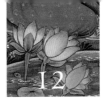

A few months after my Catholic confirmation, I saw

a flier at the yoga center after class, advertising an

upcoming yoga retreat at an ashram in Upstate

New York. I was intrigued because I was studying

Hinduism, Buddhism, and Confucianism compara-

tively at school at that time. I decided to sign up,

and together with a friend, ventured there for a

weekend in early summer.

An ashram is typically the residence of a Hindu

religious community and its guru. The guru traditionally has served as an interlocutor or conduit to God. In the Sanskrit language, the word *guru* means "one who brings lightness to the dark," meaning "he who brings knowledge to ignorance." The guru is generally one who has dedicated his life to the practice and teachings of scriptural study. He is a guide for disciples committed to a spiritual path.

This particular ashram had lost its guru in recent years. Ananda ashram now had a sort of run-down quality in his absence. It had been the home of my yoga teacher's guru since the early 1970s. Photographs of him were displayed around the rooms of a rustic country home, which had been converted into a spiritual center of sorts. He was believed to have gone on to samadhi, the enlightened state and ultimate goal of yogic practices.

We spent the next few days waking early and practicing asanas for a few hours before a vegetarian breakfast of fruit and cereals and a brief rest period before Sanskrit lessons. After lunch, there was another rest period before another afternoon asana class, then it was time for dinner. After dinner there was *satsang*, a dharma talk or spiritual lesson, followed by a group chanting sing-along. There were a few yoga teacher/musicians present who sat on the floor in front of us to lead the chants. At the end, there was a long silent meditation, then it was time for bed.

At the end of three days at Ananda, my friend invited me to drive a bit farther upstate to visit the Shree Muktananda Siddha Yoga Ashram in nearby South Fallsburg. I wanted to get the feel of another kind of ashram, this one enormously popular, thus well-funded and taken care of. Having known of Gurumayi, the female guru and descendant of the Siddha Yoga lineage, for years, and after the practices of this weekend's retreat, I felt primed for a visit.

Gurumayi is an extremely beautiful and alluring woman in her mid-forties. She looks ageless at times and slightly androgynous, too, which makes her appealing to anyone. When we arrived, the juxtaposition from Ananda was astounding. The guru was traveling. In fact, she had not been here for a year, but there was still plenty of activity without her. We checked in at a reservations desk in a large lobby, and were given name tags before we set out on a tour of the grounds.

Shree Muktananda looked and felt more like an Ivy League university campus than the modest ashram we had come from. Cafeterias, guest accommodations, bookshops, and temples were clustered together across several square miles. There was an enormous man-made lake in the center of the property with a small bridge over a narrow stream, across which the main *mandap*, or hall, and a temple were located. Statues of Shaivite deities such as Lord Shiva himself, and his warrior child, the elephant god, Ganesh, presided over the gardens. Inside, photographs of Gurumayi and other descendants, as well as colorful paintings of gods and their consorts, such as Lakshmi, the goddess of abundance, and mythological scenes from the Bhagavad Gita, decorated the numerous corridors.

On the way over to the main temple, I noticed a small garden off the walking path filled with Christian statuary. Saint Francis, the Virgin

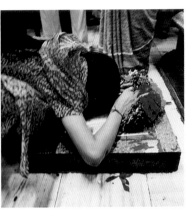

WOMAN PRESSING HER HEAD TO A PAIR OF SILVER PADAS (FEET) AT SHRINE OF SAIBABA OF SHIRDI

Mary, and Christ stood peacefully amongst tall trees with benches reserved nearby for contemplation. In the Eastern tradition, offerings of flowers and candles are offered to deities, and likewise, had been placed at their feet here. Feet are especially sacred in Hinduism and Buddhism because they represent following the footsteps of a realized being. Buddha himself is often recognized from a pair of feet rather than an image. Mary Magdalene symbolically washes the feet of the crucified Christ with her long hair, signifying the sacrifice He made of His life for our benefit. Being Catholic, and still unsure about whether being here conflicted with my own beliefs or not, I felt somewhat relieved to see these figures here.

Everyone seemed friendly and welcoming. Men and women of all ethnicities and ages moved easily through the halls, dressed conservatively and carrying books or journals. We visited Baba Nityananda's temple located in an octagon-shaped glass building with a giant bronze statue of Sri Nityananda seated in the center of the room. Many Eastern religions worship their teachers, be they family members or gurus. Nityananda was the guru of Muktananda, and Muktananda the guru of Gurumayi.

We found a seat on the floor and followed along with the *arati,* the evening chant, as the sun began to set. A golden light shed over the temple and reflected off the Nityananda *murti,* lifelike statue, as we sang. I didn't understand what I was reading along with, but I noticed a considerable improvement in my ability to pronounce the long Sanskrit words after the past weekend's retreat we had just come from. I couldn't help but compare the two ashrams, and immediately likened them to the differences between the Catholic and Protestant churches I had studied and visited. This ashram was like the Vatican of ashrams, and I could see how it might be an easy target of criticism for its opulence. However, the mood, or *bhav,* was exalted in its beauty.

I was in a new head space following the retreat. I was attempting to refrain from passing judgment on anything if I could help it.

Many Eastern religions tend to concentrate more on the experiential than the intellectual. This is a Western phenomenon, and it's a serious challenge to get out of this ingrained behavior. When we truly experience something, an inner core connection is made. This is a more holistic feeling because it involves all parts of ourselves rather than just the mind, as when we approach things intellectually. *Mana* is a word in Sanskrit that has struck me because it means, literally, "mind-heart." In the West, we tend to think of these two as opposing, even conflicting at times, but they are in essence intrinsically connected, nondualistic by nature. If we view the inner components of ourselves as dualistic, how can we not be expected to experience everything outside of ourselves in the same way?

Over dinner in one of the canteens, my friend and I decided to spend the night and head home early in the morning after reciting the "GuruGita." We had a long drive back to the city and I had class in the morning, but the energy here was charged and I felt compelled to stay overnight. The "GuruGita" is the Siddha Yoga chanting bible. It is an ode to the guru, and also a tool to bring clarity to the self through the heart by virtue of the chanting. We checked in to a double room and awoke a few hours later at 4:00 A.M. to walk through the darkness to reach the temple.

When we entered the central corridor, the sweet smell of cardamom and warmed milk from the *chai*, spiced black tea, wakened our senses. After a quick cup, we found a seat on the floor in the large carpeted auditorium. At the front of the room was the empty seat of the guru with a large photo above it; the sweet face of Swami Muktananda smiled down upon us. He was dressed in saffron-colored robes, which signified that he was a swami or religious teacher. The lulling music of the tamboura and the call of the drums enveloped us as we took our seats in lotus position and began to sway to the beat. We alternated verses with the men, who were seated across a walkway leading up to the guru's seat.

The separation of the sexes struck me as odd at first, but the effect of alternating tones was incredibly melodious. There were translations below each verse, which I tried to speed-read while at the same time trying to get the Sanskrit pronunciation and rhythm of the chant right,

too. Nearly an hour later when we were finished, we stood up to chant "Om Namah Shivaya," which means, "The divinity in me bows to honor the divinity in you." After a delicious breakfast of scrambled tofu, we started out on the road and headed back to Manhattan. I felt energized and exhausted at the same time, with so much to process and just sit with once I got home.

A group of girlfriends and I returned a month later to attend a "Satellite Intensive" at the Shree Muktananda ashram. These chanting and meditation workshops were led by Gurumayi herself, and were broadcast live around the globe to the extended Siddha Yoga community. The evening before the first day of the intensive, there was an orientation in the auditorium where newcomers and *devotees*, Siddha Yoga practitioners, could ask questions in preparation for the program. I didn't ask any questions, but listened intently to the fascinating stories of a variety of people's *shaktipat* experiences. Shaktipat is what Siddha yogis call the awakening experience that can initiate the individual into their *sadhana*, the spiritual path. Several people shared their stories of meditating or chanting to the point of ecstasy. As I lay awake that night, too excited to sleep, I set my intention to remain open to whatever experience I was ready for. I decided that if the only thing I gained from the experience was improving my meditation practice, I would have gained plenty.

The alarm went off at 4:30 A.M. and the four of us took our turns showering and dressing in the dark dormlike room. We were joined by hundreds of others as we arrived in the mandap and quietly went to our preassigned seats on the floor. We arrived early to chant the "GuruGita" in preparation for the day ahead. We broke for breakfast before the intensive began. It was as smooth and professional a production as I have seen. Devotees offered their professional services in *seva,* a donation of selfless service, for the intensive. A Boston-based newscaster served as the emcee. A large screen displayed an edited video montage about Siddha Yoga and its gurus over the years, leading us to the present day and Gurumayi's induction.

Throughout the day, there were dharma teachings given by Western Siddha Yoga Swamis. We contemplated the teachings and were led in long meditations. Sitting in an upright seated position for these long stretches was incredibly physically trying, but all a part of the practice of meditation. After all, the goal of meditation is to overcome the obstacles of everything, including the distractions caused by our very own bodies, in order to still the fluctuations of the mind.

I looked toward the empty seat of the guru all morning with the anticipation of her scheduled arrival, but as the day wore on, her absence apparent, I lost interest in all my earlier external fixations. With each meditation, I felt myself go deeper. I was beginning to understand the point of the practice, and to relish each opportunity for internal exploration. My thoughts went from the complex to the mundane, but I was able to witness them without holding on to them. It was like cleaning house in some way, because I was able to loosen the grip I held on so many unsolvable and uncontrollable situations in my life. It felt good to relinquish some responsibility, finally.

After the final afternoon break, I was resting in my spot waiting for the program to begin again when I smelled the sweet aroma of jasmine come wafting through the air. It brought a smile to my lips, and I opened my eyes knowingly and found the guru sitting in her chair, all aglow in her saffron robes, seated effortlessly in lotus position. She was looking directly in front of her with a soft smile and purposeful gaze. The room was abuzz; people rushed to their seats like schoolchildren at an assembly. The music began and Gurumayi chanted into a microphone as we responded back the same words. "Om Namoh Bhagavate Muktanandaya," she chanted to her guru, as we chanted back to her. The chant started out slowly, but came to a crescendo after fifteen minutes or so. Then everyone was silent and we all meditated for thirty minutes.

Going into meditation practice with the guru's guidance was an entirely new experience. In my meditation, I came to understand the purpose of the guru/disciple relationship for the first time. The guru can serve us as a reflection of our truest and most elevated selves. She is the projection of our divine natures, and we are hers. The guru is a living metaphor for the relationship between God and man. We are non-dualistic. We are all expressions of the

other. When it was time to open our eyes again, she was gone. Was she ever there?

We were all reeling with excitement, and shared our stories and revelations with one another animatedly over dinner that evening. We were tired and energized at once, and struggled to get to sleep again, despite obvious fatigue. In a few hours, we would start another day. We all looked forward to more self-discovery. The ashram now had a sort of utopian quality about it. It was full of spiritual study and exchange. Everyone was beaming outwardly. Glowing from within, we were lit in our hearts.

It was more challenging to remain on this spiritual path when I was back home and distractions were everywhere once again. I was changed, but it would take some work to stick to my path. I continued to go to church and to yoga class, finding that every experience was deeper. I felt things on another level, and was able to see things more clearly. Everything I read had an underlying spiritual message of truth that I recognized immediately. There was a lesson in every exchange, and I felt incredibly inspired by everything and everyone

I came into contact with. It seemed there was no limit to all I could do and be.

✦

IT HAD BEEN a year since my father's death, and I felt more awake and alive than ever before. My family and I rented a house in Tuscany for a month in the summer of 1998 in commemoration of Dad's passing. When I returned to New York, I went upstate again to take a week-long course.

I felt that I was at a critical point in my life. I was still in my static relationship, and I was nearing my thirtieth birthday and graduation. What would I do with my life? I was far closer to myself now, but what did my future hold? It seemed as though I had more options than ever before, but I felt I had to be certain when I took that first step, because I was starting off older than my peers at school. In this silent retreat, I was intent on determining the course for the next chapter of my life. Each day, I asked for clarity in meditation. "Let go, let go," was my preferred mantra. Let go of the past and embrace the future. I left the retreat more clear than when I entered, but the answers did not fall into my lap. Or, maybe I

was not ready to deal with the truth. At least I was another step closer to myself, and ready for the year ahead. I was twenty-nine when I began my final year of college in the fall of 1998, and would turn thirty in January.

There was a Siddha Yoga winter retreat being held in Northern California, not far from where I grew up. I invited my mother to join me there for my birthday. I was the age that she had been when she had given birth to me thirty years before. We ventured to Santa Clara, and roomed together in a convention center hotel just off the highway. My mother had been intrigued by my recent fascinations with the spiritual realm, and seemed thrilled that I had chosen her to spend my birthday with. I talked her through various aspects of yoga that were now familiar to me, but left some things for her own discovery through observation and experience. She joined me in chanting the "GuruGita" early in the mornings, and in volunteering to help serve others in the breakfast queue in the cafeteria. She sat by my side in meditation, cross-legged on the floor for hours at a time without complaint. I was happy to share this with someone who appreciated it as much as I did. Finally, we had something to share together again.

Bakasana
(crane or crow pose)

Baka means "crane." Like kukkutasana, the hands and arms support the weight of the body in this posture. Bakasana is said to resemble a crane wading in water.

Throughout history, the crane has symbolized a herald of death and war as well as, in Christianity, a symbol for vigilance and goodness. In Eastern symbolism, the crane is often said to represent long life. The crane posture is good for strengthening the arms and wrists, as well as stretching the back, strengthening the abdominal organs, and opening the groin.

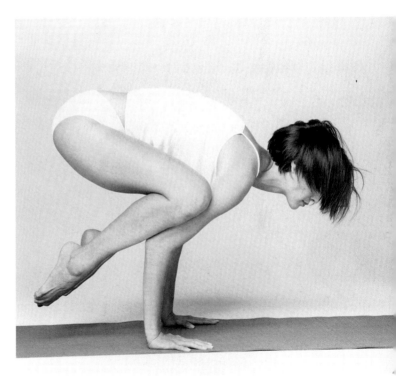

COMMUNITY

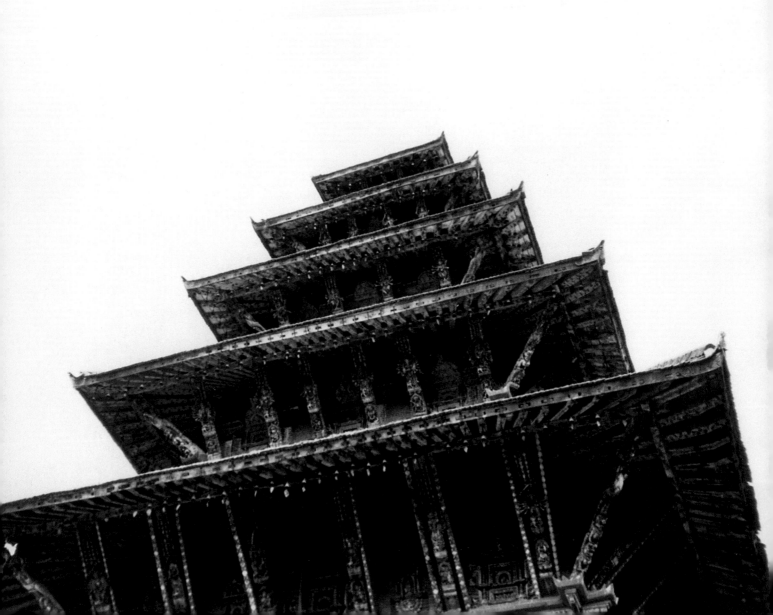

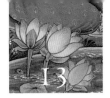

13

Many institutions were created from communities of like-mindedness, each designed to create order and provide answers during otherwise chaotic times. For centuries, the intentions of various communities, from religion to government, have served well for many in offering comfort and security, but they have also shut out many who do not quite fit their expected molds. From this is born intolerance, which breeds hatred in the world. Today, more and more, the world seems made up of too many alternative and opposing communities. We can easily forget that there is a place for everyone, something for everybody; and we can easily get caught up in fanatical solidarity, which creates too great a disconnect from what is seemingly "other."

The word *community* is derived from the Latin word *comunitas*. *The American Heritage Dictionary* defines community as (1) a group of people living in the same locality and under the same government; (2) a group of people having common interests; (3) society as a whole. Looking at the latter, we must consider our knowledge that humans are social animals and require interaction with others. More than anything, we need love, understanding, and respect, which to a certain extent we can provide for ourselves if we so choose. But, clichéd as it may sound, no one is an island. Though it is always a good idea to begin with what we have some control over in life, rather than those things outside of ourselves that we have little to no control over anyway, our end goal should be uniting with others, as this leads us back to creation. For individuals cannot survive alone. It is only in relationships that indi-

viduals can fulfill their potential and truly be themselves. A true community must not only be inclusive and provide comfort to those who choose to enter it; those in it must *feel* it. As people choose to change, that which is outside of their own community is a major influence on their individual decisions.

When I think of the word *community*, I think of the word *commune*, which means to experience heightened receptivity. When we come together or work together, we can achieve so much more than we can independently. We form our communities from these two needs—the need for self-determination and the need for one another.

In the course of our lives, there are numerous sub-communities that we will enter and perhaps even leave. The family is the first of these experiences, which no longer must adhere to traditional definitions, but is a constantly evolving notion and is by far the most vital, as it has a powerful influence over an individual's thoughts and value system. Whether the family has one or fifteen members, if we are to completely embrace the progress of thinking, we then must embrace the evolution of definitions. Most importantly, if there is love within the family, the child will have a greater chance of loving herself and others throughout her life.

Another sub-community experience is school, which also has come to mean a variety of things. There are private and public schools, as well as home-schooling, which is gaining in popularity. We can even consider a group or collective of independent thinkers, artists, or individuals with a common cause a community. This is where many of us first realize that we share a sameness with our peers, while maintaining our uniquely different personalities. Church and temple are, for many of us, a community as well. They should be an extension of human values, which can be referred to as family values, but also a context for history, which should also be explored through education and questioned through experience. Each community must value tolerance above all else. Who was it who said "Ignorance is bliss"? I would say that ignorance is death.

As we mature, we are often faced with con-flicting ideas such as the absolute need for individual freedom and the unequivocal need for relationships. In nature, successful examples of this paradox abound, and reveal surprising treasures of insight. The real challenge is to really be tolerant, in both thought and action, even when very committed to our ideas and beliefs. If our faith is strong, we should be all the more accepting of another's faith. Though it may sound idealistic, it is possible to create communities that thrive in paradox. If we were to view this world as it truly is—a macrocosm—then we would understand that we all have a place and purpose within it. We are all parts of a sum. If we get too consumed by the micro, we can't experience the beauty and peace that exists in the macro.

So many of the world's current problems are rooted in these supposed differences, and we stand divided by man-made concepts of separation. No matter what our beliefs, we all understand that we come from somewhere. Whether you believe it was through an immaculate conception or the big bang, we were born together into humanity. We inherited life and the capacity to be humane, which allows us to experience life fully and with God's grace. Belonging together is defined by a shared sense of purpose, not by shared beliefs about specific behaviors. The instinct of community is everywhere in life. Life is systems-seeking; it instinctively needs to be in relationships, to be connected to others. It is possible to create resilient and adaptive communities that welcome our diversity as well as our membership. Let us choose togetherness, and embrace otherness.

IMPERMANENCE

"Impermanent are all Created Things. Strive on Mindfully."
—BUDDHA

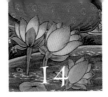

14

September 11, 2001, was a historic day for the entire world. Those of us who were in New York had prime seats in witnessing humanity under the threat of terrorism as the World Trade Center virtually dissolved under attack before our very eyes. Horrid as these events were, in their aftermath we have come together in mourning and in fear as a community and nation as a whole. As many of us question the existence of a God who could allow such evil and hatred in the world in His name, others experience solidarity for the first time among family members, business colleagues, our government, and the rest of the free world, while others still witness all as the play of consciousness.

At the time, over 5,000 bodies had not yet been accounted for, leaving thousands upon thousands behind without closure. Our president and his cabinet were deciding what our retaliation would be against those to whom we had appointed the responsibility for these barbaric acts. In life there are always choices, and the choice then seemed to be either in battling the enemy eye for eye, or in collectively finding a way to channel our grief and anger in a more mindful way. Can we consciously risk more human lives to gain justice for those lost?

Yogically speaking, we have all lived this scenario before many times over throughout the world's history. This is the way tragedies are thus explained in ancient texts like the Bhagavad Gita. Lives are lost so that new lives can be born. There is no final death as such. The cycle continues: death, birth, death, birth, and so on. Each life has a specific purpose, and terminates when that divinely predestined

point is reached. Parts of ourselves die each day, and in each death of another, we are reminded of our own fates. When we mourn, we mourn ourselves along with those we lose. When we reach the state of samadhi, we reunite with our source. This and moksha (liberation) are the goals for Hindus. We all die in tragedies of this magnitude, but we also survive and carry on with the memories and teachings of those gone ahead, as well.

It is valuable to look at how various religions deal with death and retribution. For Christians, Christ's life teaches his followers through his own unjust and cruel death inflicted on the cross, which he experienced for the good of us all, so that we could learn that we, too, can rise up if we maintain our faith in God and in the afterlife. For Muslims, the Koran says that if a man kills an innocent person, to God it looks as if he is killing all innocent people on earth; and that if you save an innocent person, it looks to God as if you are saving all innocent people on earth.

Buddhism explains this through the teachings and life of Gautama Buddha, who had four sightings on secret trips outside his palace walls, which led to his enlightenment. On the first trip, he meets an old man; on the second, he sees a very sick man. On the third venture, he sees a corpse being carried to a crematory; and on the fourth, he comes across a sadhu (holy man) or renunciate. The cumulative effects of these encounters are traumatic to Buddha, but he realizes through them the truth about the human condition; that all human beings are susceptible to sickness, old age, and death. Having witnessed all of this, he matures very quickly and with new clarity. He then focuses only on the important questions or issues regarding life. The last sighting of the holy man awakens Buddha's dormant spirituality when he recognizes that this man with nothing has such tranquility and peace about him. He spends the next several years in seeking a solution to the problem of human suffering.

Let us follow in Buddha's footsteps in the aftermath of these and all tragedies. We need to view the world with new clarity, and to focus on the important questions or issues regarding life. Allow this experience to awaken our dormant spirituality and seek tranquility and peace. Let us embrace Buddha's last words before dying: "Impermanent are all created things. Strive on mindfully."

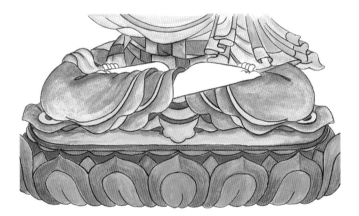

Eka Pada Rajakapotasana
(king pigeon pose)

Eka means "one," *pada* means "leg" or "foot," and *kapota*, "pigeon." Another difficult back-bending posture, eka pada rajakapotasana imitates the king pigeon's puffed

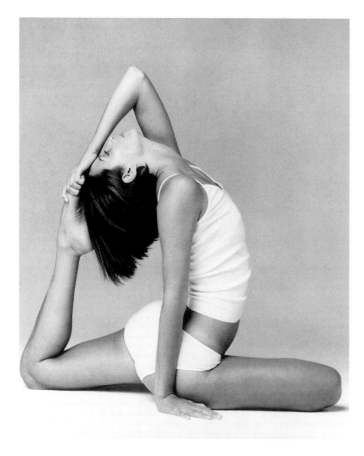

chest. Part of the difficulty of this posture is the positioning of the legs. As a result of the complexity, it is difficult to achieve proper balance and pelvic alignment, making even movement along the spine and sacrum quite challenging. With one leg kneeling and the other bent in front, this posture is also beneficial to the lower spine, the pelvis, and the urinary system. The opening of the various parts of the body, from the pelvis to the shoulder muscles, provides a fresh supply of blood to the endocrine glands. This posture also works the shoulders and neck to relieve stiffness.

Urdhva Dhanurasana
(upward bow pose or wheel)

This posture essentially imitates a back-bend. Part of the practice of yoga is to offer the practitioner different views and perspectives, both of the body and of the mind. Just as sarvangasana and salamba sirsasana force the body upside down and invert one's perspective, urdhva dhanurasana shifts one's perspective from the front of the body to the back of the body. Moving from the front of the body to the more unfamiliar back of the body, the back-bend requires an entire mental and physical focus shift into the back. In urdhva dhanurasana, it is important to maintain passivity and relaxation in the muscles of the front part of the body, such as the groin and abdominal and chest muscles. This pose greatly stretches the chest and lungs, while strengthening the arms, wrists, abdomen, legs, buttocks, and spine. It also opens up the chest and lungs, and stimulates the pituitary and thyroid, resulting in feelings of vitality and energy. Urdhva dhanurasana is a good pose to counteract depression and relieve back pain, and is therapeutic for both asthma and osteoporosis.

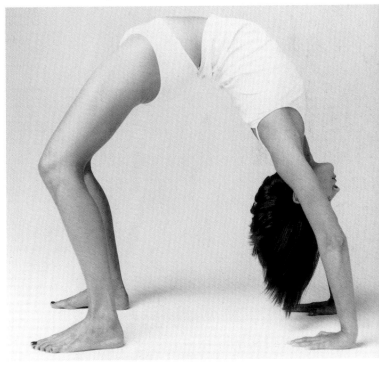

DHARMA (TEACHINGS)

Be a Lamp Unto Yourself

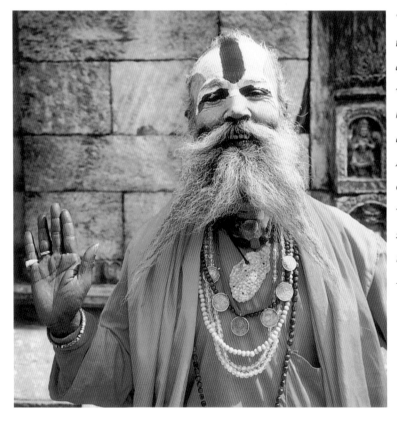

"We seek gurus because we want someone to show us who we are. This notion is an absurdity. We live within the sphere of our vanities—our own lusts, brutalities, habits, attachments, and anxieties. These are all that we know; they are our life. And as long as we are looking to someone, or something else for the truth of ourselves, we cannot look at this sphere of our self—and thus we will never see who we truly are."

—JOHN McAFEE

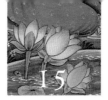
The tendency is easy. We all have it to some

degree—knowing what issues we each have to over-

come, and wishing that someone or something could

simply lift them away in one single swoop. We can

certainly be assisted on our journeys, both spiritual

and otherwise, throughout our lives, but we all know

that we must experience things for ourselves if we are

to truly learn anything. Self-realization is just that,

self-realization. Guidance should be welcomed, but

not without some ringing of truth within us. Not everything we are taught is always appropriate for us.

Many people in the East, and even in the West, claim to have gurus. The word is so popular today that many people misuse it without knowing what it really means or implies. It is used so much, in fact, that it has become a loose metaphor for a teacher of any kind. *Guru* is actually another Sanskrit word, which means "to bring light to darkness." Darkness, in this case, refers to ignorance or the delusion of reality. The guru is traditionally a bestower of great wisdom; someone who has achieved an enlightened state of being through mastering the eight limbs of yoga.

Buddha was himself enlightened, and was a great guru. He was a walking, talking, living example that these yogic practices could lead other human beings to the liberated state he had reached within his own lifetime. His path was a practical one, and thus began what evolved into one of today's quickest growing philosophical religions in the world. He taught this path in his own terms through the Four Noble Truths and the Eightfold Path

throughout his entire life so that others, too, could experience bliss. After all, each of us carries the potential for enlightenment, in much the same way an apple seed carries the potential to be an apple tree.

Like the Buddha, those who have experienced awakening may continue to study and teach by example to whomever they may attract. In India, where the Buddha was born, gurus are abundant. In fact, some yogis may have more than just one guru or spiritual teacher. There are many ways in which the relationships with gurus are formed and maintained. I have friends who say that they dreamed of their guru from their home in the United States, and then traveled all the way to India in search of him. Some continue to mourn long after their guru has left his body. And, while I have spent some time around a few gurus in the past few years and have closely observed them with their audiences in an effort to better understand the relationship, I have not been compelled to call any contemporary teachers "my guru." I have, however, many times been inspired by the truth and knowledge that comes through these individuals who seem to hold a certain power in their wisdom, which is believed to be passed through a kind of grace through them and onto others by their actions and words, or even merely by their presence. Although, growing up Catholic, and therefore Christian, I have naturally considered Jesus Christ as my guide. Each time that I write my name, I am reminded of His significance in the world and in my life. I guess I could consider Him my first guru.

Traditionally, the role of the guru is held by men, and is passed down through one kind of lineage or another. It is widely believed that their knowledge can also be bestowed or transferred onto another being when one leaves his physical body or dies, as in the Siddha Yoga lineage where Gurumayi is the figurehead of their ashrams around the world. In India, it is the guru's function to preside over an ashram and share his knowledge on the various teachings with his devotees.

Devotees are the disciples or students, and also sometimes the caretakers of the guru and the ashram. Devotees often serve their gurus as though they were a deity, as they are believed to be closer to God than most because of their heightened awareness. Dharma, meant to represent truth itself, is bestowed upon devotees, as well as any other teachings that will help them realize this truth within their lives and within themselves as they sit adjacent to the guru as he speaks to them.

Today, there are several well-known female gurus as well, such as Gurumayi, Mother Meera, Ananda Ma, and Amma, also known as the hugging guru. These world-renowned gurus can speak at once to audiences of hundreds at any given time or when touring the world, as many of them often do. In these situations, it is nearly impossible to reach the level of intimacy that was traditionally once typical of a guru's audience. Knowledge can still be shared and closeness still felt, but it is much harder to directly access mentoring when on these foreign tours than that which still occurs more easily in India, where the relationship was first established.

One of the most beautiful things I have noticed with regards to the traditions of gurus is that each guru has a guru himself or herself, and those gurus are regarded as highly as their devotees regard them. This gives a sense that each one of us is a teacher and a

Tantric Buddhism, otherwise known as *Vajrayana,* or the diamond way, an esoteric tradition of Buddhism, "depends heavily on direct initiation or 'empowerment' by a guru," and should only be properly practiced under the close guidance of a spiritual teacher.

Kashmir Shaivism is a Hindu practice that also relies heavily on the initiation by a guru. Siddha Yoga is an example of this form of worship, initiated by the guru's grace, which teaches that divine consciousness is attainable within the body.

Tantra

In Sanskrit, *Tantra* translates as "techniques" and originates from the early part of the first millennium from texts known as the Tantras. Their teachings are dedicated to the principle of shakti, or the body's primordial energy, which, when dormant and as an obstacle to the flow of prana, can be awakened through a practice based on kundalini. Tantric Yoga, specifically Hindu Tantra, emphasizes a practice whose goal is to integrate the self with the Self, as well as the physical body with the spiritual cosmos, through using certain energies that are usually encouraged to be relinquished, such as sexual pleasure, to reduce obstacles that block prana.

student at the same time. There is another kind of guru called an "upaguru," who can be anyone who teaches you. Humility is an important factor in a teacher, and wisdom is not something that should merely feed the self-righteous ego. On the contrary, these characteristics are to be shared with others or deeply contemplated for yourself. Misusing one's knowledge or wrongly guiding another vulnerable soul under spiritual pretenses is a heinous act that will surely have reciprocally fitting karmic implications. For a bhakti yogi, the guru is indispensable, while he is often an obstacle for a jnana yogi. Therefore, we must heed what we know and, in addition, seek guidance from another.

You should be aware of these facts as you explore or enter into the new world of yoga. Ego is a powerful condition, and counterproductive to yogic aspirations, which may still exist even in longtime practitioners. Beware of those who claim to know more than you do. Again, trust your instincts and your experience above all else as you make your way through this world. Many of us teach what we most need to learn in life. Projection can be a common side effect, but it should be avoided at all costs.

Even in asana class, for instance, it is important to listen to our own bodies. Due to increasing popularity, yoga classes are often very full. It is often difficult for a teacher to give you the individualized kind of care you may require, so it is incredibly important to be aware of your own body at all times. Don't always try to go 100 percent in a posture that you are not familiar with. Go slowly and take it easy. Check in with yourself at every point and with every breath. It is more important to be aligned properly than to reach the final posture; proper alignment will protect you. The Buddha once said, "Be a lamp unto yourself." This is excellent advice, and worth reminding yourself of frequently as you walk this path.

Ustrasana
(camel pose)

Most of our daily tasks involve motions that bend the body in a forward direction, stretching the posterior side of the spine. It is rare that we counteract such

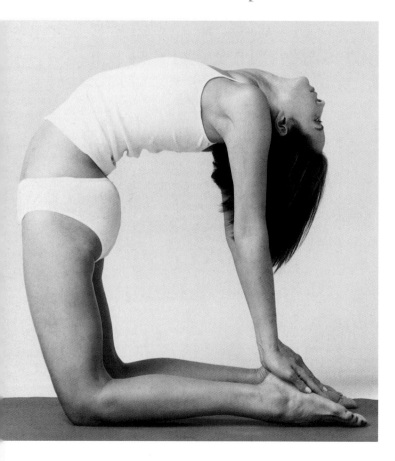

motions by bending the other way. However, it is very important to stretch the spinal column in a concave movement, as extending the anterior spine helps blood circulation. Performing backbends, in a number of variations of postures, opens the chest and energizes the lungs, deepening breathing and allowing more oxygenated blood to freely circulate throughout the entire body. One of these postures is ustrasana, or camel posture.

This posture is called the camel posture because it is said to resemble the shape of the camel. The meanings of the asanas are often suggested by their names, and those named after animals hold some of the more interesting parallels. As the camel's poor eyesight pushes the animal to rely on some inner compass to navigate its way through the inhospitable climate of the desert, so does this posture require one to consider another way of seeing. The shape of this posture places one's head and vision behind the body. As in the sirsasana, our world is turned upside down and our perspective inverted. With the change of our everyday, forward-facing vision, we can cultivate a more important inner vision. The back-bend itself presents a challenging and less-than-hospitable environment for the body. But when developed and practiced properly, ustrasana fosters balance and strengthens the spine. This posture simultaneously opens the chest and pelvis, promotes flexibility in the shoulders, and stretches and tones the lower abdominals and quadriceps.

Kapotasana
(pigeon pose)

Kapota means "pigeon." This is a more advanced back-bend that imitates the shape of the pigeon. It tones the entire spine through circulating blood around the

spinal column, opens the chest and pelvis, and strengthens the heart and abdominals. It is essential to master kapotasana before practicing more difficult back-bending postures.

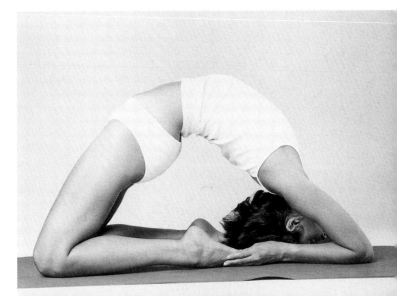

BEAUTY IS IN THE HEART OF THE BEHELD

"Everything has beauty, but not everyone sees it."
—CONFUCIUS

16

Writing about beauty is a challenge for me. Not

because I don't have an opinion about it, but because

I have made a career out of being perceived as "beau-

tiful." I have allowed myself to be a marketing tool

and a seller of "beautiful" things. As a model, it feels

narcissistic to even contemplate this. And as a

woman, it is also difficult, as we often allow ourselves

to fall victim to societal notions. But yoga has taught

me another thing—that health and well-being are

where true beauty lies in terms of the physical, nothing more and nothing less. When it comes to the spirit, there are endless expressions of beauty. You can find the beauty in everything once you start to recognize God's hand or the power of nature in its creation. However, in order to appreciate beauty on this level, our perceptions must first change.

As children, we respond to beauty instinctually, before we even put into order our emotions and thoughts. But, as we mature and become exposed to others and the world at large, our conception of beauty shifts from an internal experience or intuitive response to an outward experience or reaction to stimuli. We begin to create our own self-images by comparing ourselves with those around us, or with the inexhaustible inundation of images in our culture. My career aside, I grew up like every other little girl in that it felt like an overnight experience when I became aware of my physical person. The "comparing" started earlier than that, though. Naturally, I was comparing myself to my parents or siblings early on, and as the middle of three daughters, I would gauge myself by my sisters on either side, hardly conscious of what I was doing. I finally

became aware that I was doing this when I reached prepubescence. I caught myself comparing most often when I was among my peers at school or while playing team sports. By this time your family has become familiar enough to you but, by contrast, your friends and their families suddenly seem utterly intriguing.

At that age, there was always something your best friend had that you didn't have but really wanted: such as a mom who spoiled you by taking you for ice cream after school or the big brother who looked after you on the playground. Those differences may have even been what brought you and your best friend together. As human beings, we have always been inclined to seek out what we don't have and to try to alter what we do have in order to feel more comfortable in life. I had curly brown hair and was always taller than every other girl in my class. I had lots of friends who were very small, with straight light hair. I liked their compactness and cuteness. They had an easier time than me finding clothes that complemented their figures, plus my height and my features made me appear older than I was, which made people treat me differently, whether or not I wanted it. I often imagined myself sticking out like a sore thumb. I began to slump my shoulders and slouch in order to make myself appear smaller so that I would fit in amongst my circle of friends. This was the early formation of the self-image of myself that would stay with me into adulthood, as it will if you are not conscious of it.

My mother was petite, too. We were the same height when I was ten, and I could fit into most of her clothes. I suppose there were advantages—the fact that many girls want to appear older most of the time, for instance—but with it came an early sense of responsibility. Whether in class or on the softball field, adults seemed to expect more from me because of my size. They talked to me differently than to the others. When getting reprimanded, I always seemed to receive more "warning" by eye contact. As a result, I came to expect more from myself, too.

When I was ten, my dad's job relocated us to Miami. This is where I was "discovered." My sister and I both showed horses, something we had begun to do in California but became more serious about in Florida. One day after school, as we were having a lesson with our trainer, a photographer showed up with subjects to shoot around the stables. I felt his eyes fixating on me as I trotted around the ring on my horse, Dewey. I was fourteen.

I loved riding more than anything else, and absolutely enjoyed practicing because I was so committed. It was a labor of love. So, when that photographer saw me riding my horse, he was seeing me at my best and most confident, and he found me to be beautiful. I don't recall that I had ever been told that I was beautiful before. He asked both my sister and me if he could take our pictures. We asked our mother for permission, and she agreed. She brought us to his home studio one Saturday morning where we spent the day getting our makeup done by the photographer's wife and having our pictures taken.

My sister was indeed beautiful and naturally athletic, and she was aware of it, too. Everybody treated her specially because she seemed so, well, perfect. She was two years older than me—a critical difference in age at that time in your life—and she was incredibly confident in her body, whereas I was not.

At fourteen, I was five foot eight and all legs. I had braces, too. I was at that "awkward stage" that people talk about, and I had very little confidence in my physical being. Fortunately, some of my friends were also going through that stage, so I wasn't completely alone. I was always pretty social, too, so my friendships gave me some joy during that self-conscious time.

I was truly surprised later when the photographer seemed so pleased with the results of our shoot. He contacted a local agent and immediately set up an appointment for us with the agency's owner. My mom drove us and accompanied us as our photos were inspected and as we sat by quietly and uncomfortably waiting for the scrutinizing agent to deliver her verdict. Finally, after several minutes of hemming and hawing, the skinny woman with dark hair and sharp features squinted at us through serious black-rimmed glasses and told our mother that my sister was too short but that I would be able to find some work. At that moment, I wanted nothing more than to trade legs with my sister so that she could find work as a model, not me. But that, obviously, was not a possibility.

Here I was, fourteen, thrust into the "world of beauty" before I myself even had any sense of my place within that context. I went from cleaning stalls at the barn for five dollars a stall, making at the most twenty-five dollars a day or fifty dollars a weekend, to making sixty dollars an hour! My mom drove me to all of my appointments and bookings after school for the next year. She would sit waiting for me while I worked. It was strange work, right from the start. I was paid an hourly rate that started as soon as I walked into the studio. I would sit while my makeup and hair were done, then dress and step in front of the camera. I always say now that modeling isn't a craft like acting, for example, because you never really receive any formal training, but, in actuality, there is a sort of on-the-job training that comes with practice and through experience. Until then, I always felt really self-conscious, but as the photographers and clients were constantly so complimentary, I slowly began to relax.

Surprisingly, other teenaged models with more experience proved to be great teachers. I remember one girl in particular whose name was Natalie. She was also a dancer, and seemed really mature compared to me. She was elegant in her movements and incredibly professional. Whether we were working together or in a group, she would act out scenarios to make her roles look more believable in the photos. I learned a lot quickly from Natalie through imitation.

I soon started to build a clientele and was working pretty regularly. When my family decided to move back to California following my dad's heart attack, I was sad to leave some of the friends I had made. Though I was enjoying the exposure to a new world, and also appreciative of the opportunity to make some of my own money to help out with Dewey, I sometimes missed just being a kid. Between my riding lessons, horse shows on weekends, and shoots after school, I had little time for my friends or for fun.

We moved back to the same town we had lived in four years before. It was still familiar yet somehow felt changed, probably from our living elsewhere. It was strange to be back. I felt differently than how I remembered feeling when I had lived there before. We moved back in the middle of the school year, so I was the new kid coming in. I had lost touch with most of my childhood friends, and now missed those I'd left behind. My family began to settle in but I knew I never would. We brought our horses out West, but never really got into riding the way we had back in Florida.

My mom and I went to see a modeling agency in San Francisco so I could resume at least that. Soon, I was commuting from the suburbs to the city a couple of times a week to work or to go on appointments after school. Working gave me a sense of independence, which I relished more and more as I soon started to get myself to the city and back on my own. I would take a bus to the train and then ride the train into downtown, from where I would then either walk or take a cab to my destination. It was not at all difficult to find this new lifestyle more exciting than school, but it took a toll on my studies as a result.

That summer, Mom and I went to Paris, the fashion capital of the world, to see what I could do. Apparently not much, but we had a great time finding our way through Paris together, just enjoying each other's company, visiting museums, and living the café life. When I returned to school that fall, I started to sow my teenage oats a bit. A typical teenager, I started to act out, along with my friends and my sisters, toward our parents and school authoritarians. My friends and I wore all black every day to school and called ourselves "mods," likening our look to beatniks and the characters in the movie *Quadrophenia*. We would visit the Berkeley campus to listen to bands, shop in thrift stores, and smoke cigarettes in coffee bars. These teenage activities grossly contradicted my work life. I chose to keep it to myself and began living a double life from then on. I was ashamed of my modeling life when I was with my friends, and embarrassed by my teenage life when I was working with the grown-ups. I guess the shame came from the fact that I was not being truthful to myself in either situation.

My body was finally developing into that of a woman, which made me very happy (although I would have preferred to have more of some things and less of others). My breasts were the last to develop, but my hips and bottom had already taken shape. People at work seemed to like my body the way it was, but at school I still felt irregularly proportioned. At sixteen, I went to New York City for the summer to model. I was now almost my full height of five

foot ten and weighed about 118 pounds. I set out on my own, but stayed with my agents in their town house on the Upper East Side. For the first few weeks, I pounded the pavement by day and had fun at night with the other teenaged girls from around the world who shared the same guardians. We went to the movies and ate pizza, comparing stories about our daytime appointments and work. It felt more like a boarding school dorm than a town house. There was little to no competition. We supported one another and commiserated together when we lost a job or missed our families or boyfriends, if there was one in the picture. I started to work regularly, and with more and more important clients, such as *Vogue* and *Elle* magazines. I continued to learn through my experiences and from the people who were surrounding me. I was a long way away from the preteen fashion section of the local newspaper's department store ads back in Miami.

In these next few years at work, I became more observant and quiet, though I was also starting to enjoy some moderate success. People were asking for me by name, and I enjoyed the recognition I sometimes received. Whatever hang-ups I had had with my body were eradicated by the constant flattery that I was hearing from makeup artists, stylists, and photographers. I knew better than to take their comments too seriously, but I couldn't help allowing it to make me feel good now and again. On the flip side, I saw lots of behavior around me that I found suspect. Many people I encountered seemed to possess those character flaws that I desperately wanted to avoid. There were those who thought too highly of themselves, and then those who didn't give themselves enough credit. Just like back home at school, amidst braces and awkward teenage moments.

I remember observing the other models, especially the European girls who seemed so comfortable with their bodies, studying them like a bird-watcher. Walking around the dressing rooms in the nude seemed like second nature to them. Sometimes, I tried to emulate them. It didn't always work. I never felt totally comfortable, though nobody seemed to notice. I would sit there smoking, as if I were doing something purposeful, pretending to be grown-up, absorbing it all into my little universe within. It was truly an exciting time at the beginning. I traveled the world over, visiting all of the places I had read about in books and daydreamed about on sleepy afternoons. This wasn't such a bad way to live for a couple of years, I thought. Save some money, maybe go back to school one day. The world seemed wide open.

I turned eighteen on an airplane somewhere over the South Pacific en route to Thailand from California in 1987. I visited Phuket and Bali, as well, and then went on to another shoot in Cairo, Egypt, where we floated up the Nile to Aswan and Luxor. When I returned to New York, I was an adult and ready to move into my first apartment located downtown on the outskirts of SoHo. There was only one problem: I had yet to graduate from high school.

At that moment, I felt so far away from school. All I wanted now was to live life on my own terms and travel around the world. As simple as that. For the previous few years I had been going to an independent study school near my parents' home that allowed me to come and go as I pleased, reporting to just one advisor who then taught me in one-on-one sessions. It was a perfect solution for my ever-changing situation. My course study was designed around my travel and my interests in literature and geography.

Once I arrived in New York, as an adult, I was able to call my own shots. I began accepting constant work, right off the bat, which left little time for studying or going back to California to check in with my advisor. I was too busy running forward to catch a glimpse of what I might be leaving behind. I just left it open-ended and gave it little thought, if at all. My mother was beside herself over my indifference. She brought it up every chance she got, but I told her that it was no longer of practical use to me. It was almost too easy for me, and I couldn't see the value in continuing anymore.

After a few months on my own, living in the big city and working full-time as a model, I started to experience a change of heart. Without that other life, the one I'd practically fled, I felt less interesting and much lonelier. All around me there were these blatant examples of impermanence in everything, from "beauty," which stemmed from my career, to every other false sense of security that had thus far been afforded to me. I began to desire more for myself. I met my first serious boyfriend at that transitional point, and he introduced me to yoga. I was horrified when my mother shared my shameful secret with him—that I was essentially a high school dropout. But, it was that sense of shame and his support that ultimately made me complete my schoolwork and earn my degree in a few months' time.

Now a young woman, I spent the next few years discovering myself. I quit smoking and started eating better and exercising regularly. I took my first writing class one summer at UCLA. I was feeling healthy and stimulated. The relationship didn't work out in the end, but I was at least left with the yoga, which was there to stay in some form or another. Through yoga, I was gifted the tools to bring myself to a calmer state when necessary. The relationship had been unhealthy for me because I felt criticized by and in competition with my partner. It was empowering to leave a relationship that was not serving me, and now I was stronger on my own than I had ever been before. Before the relationship, I had bought my first apartment in New York, but had not been living there much because I had been spending a lot of time out in L.A. with my boyfriend. It felt good to be home.

At first, going back into work and traveling again seemed healing. People I had worked with warmly welcomed me back and made me feel beautiful again, for whatever it was worth. But before long I was back to old and bad habits from before—smoking, drinking more, and working too much to take care of myself. Rather than choosing to learn from my relationship and the breakup, I instead ran with the pain and anger I had accumulated. I ran for an entire year and when I felt it was finally somewhat out of my system, I stopped and I stayed. I met somebody new and began to feel more hopeful about being in a relationship again. I quit smoking for good, at last, after a few futile attempts. I stopped drinking, too, and began to exercise with regularity again.

It wasn't until I was twenty-six that I decided to return full-time to school. The decision came after feeling rejected in my new "smoke-free" body at the couture shows in Paris. I had gained roughly ten pounds, but felt good about my health and my body. To me, it was completely worth it. For the first time, though, the industry was less comfortable with my body than I was. I didn't like doing the shows much anyway, so I took the cool reception that I received as the impetus for a much-needed change. I knew that I wouldn't be happy doing this job forever, nor would this job be forever happy with me. I was already becoming bored with it much of the time, and I didn't care to be scrutinized now that I was an adult woman and more sensitive to the endless projections. I needed to challenge myself. I had often thought of returning to school, so I decided that there was no time like the present to give it a shot. This decision was cathartic for me because the commitment to my classes forced me to turn down work that required travel. It grounded me and kept me home. It felt good to finally develop a routine, to keep my refrigerator full, and to see my friends more regularly.

School gave me so much that I looked forward to every book and every class, each and every day. I still wasn't completely sure about what I was seeking from it, which didn't matter anyway because I was enjoying it so much, filling myself with knowledge, continuously stimulated. I explored every subject that I had ever expressed an interest in, the list of which seemed endless. It was a glorious time of personal growth. I came into my own during those four years. I was left alone and was able to prove myself with my knowledge rather than with my body and face. At this time, I also reconnected with a regular yoga practice. Because yoga connected my mind, body, and spirit, when my dad died, I was able to nurture myself through my grieving process and emerge from it even stronger. I learned to accept my body exactly as it was. It had brought me all this way through life, and didn't deserve the judgment and criticism that I'd exposed it to.

My height had brought me good fortune and set me apart from my sisters when I was younger. When I was modeling more frequently, my shapely hips were constant reminders of my femininity when many of the clothes I had to wear and sell were not cut for women's bodies. I was tall and thin, but never skinny. My breasts were just the right size for me and not for show, as that was not their purpose anyway. I had grown up thinking of myself as gawky and uncoordinated, and had fortunately outgrown *that*. I discovered that I could be graceful and agile and could hold my balance in challenging poses, both as a model and as a yogi. I came to love my body because it was strong, supple, and pliable, not because

of what it looked like. In yoga, I owned my body. It was so completely connected to the rest of me, and I was in control of that. Through yoga, I came to understand the metaphor of the body as a temple. It has to be strong and sturdy, but only to protect and sustain the inner workings of the heart and the mind. I could finally feel the union between mind, body, and spirit.

Our bodies deserve gratitude, not self-loathing. Each of us has her own unique set of physical assets that we can and should feel good about. If we allow our physical assets to take precedence over what is inside of us, then it is no wonder why so many of us fall into this behavior. We possess the ability within us to change that. It is so important to learn to love yourself if you do not already. We are our own authority and cannot blame others for allowing us to feel bad about ourselves. If we allow others to make us feel inferior in any way, we will put ourselves into harmful, perhaps even life-threatening, circumstances. This is not the way we attain the best from ourselves. We must be gentle, kind, and always forgiving.

This requires some unconditioning, of course,

but with practice and taking better care of ourselves, little by little, we may start to feel better. It is often harder to "unlearn" than to learn. When we feel our best, we also look our best. You can't have one without the other.

This is what I have discovered through a variety of experiences and through *Ayurveda*. Inner beauty radiates from within. Some say that beauty is in the eye of the beholder. I would say that beauty is in the heart of the beheld.

Salamba sirsasana
(supported headstand)

Consider your feet the foundation on which you stand. They are like roots that support you on the earth. At the other end of your body is the brain, the seat of *jiva*.

Jiva is life, your individual soul or essence. It is believed that to develop the jiva, one must surrender the security of the earth and uproot oneself—literally turn oneself upside down. The brain is also the controller of the intellect, the will, the memory, the imagination, and the thinking, as stated in *Yoga: A Gem for Women* by Geeta S. Iyengar. It is the center of *sattva* (like jiva, it is your essence, meaning purity, truth, lucidity), one of the three *gunas* (dynamic forces) of *prakrti* (nature, cosmic manifestation). With your feet suddenly rooted above in heaven, you become nourished spiritually and divinely. Practicing balance and courage in this position—carrying your own weight—helps you look at the weight of your burdens from a different perspective, from an unfamiliar angle.

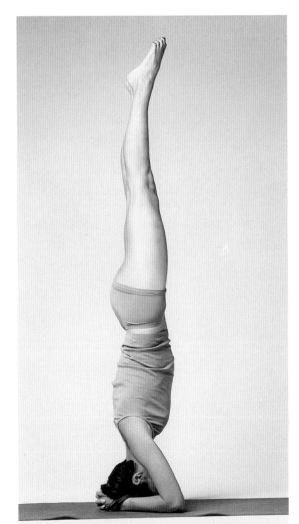

Physically, the headstand stimulates blood supply and circulation to the brain, bringing clarity of mind and speech. Head-balance revitalizes the whole body and strengthens the spine. Standing upright all of the time, the body's internal organs tend to sag with gravity and become sluggish. Practicing upside down helps to counteract these effects. With the increased blood circulation, your respiration and digestion are also improved. The most obvious effects, however, are on the brain itself. The inverted posture brings more oxygen to the brain, which increases mental sharpness and intellectual clarity. More blood flow to the brain even invigorates teeth, gums and other organs located in the head. For the practitioner, the greatest benefits are perhaps developing the strength and flexibility of the body while stimulating and disciplining the mind, all to achieve inner balance.

WHAT IS
AYURVEDA?

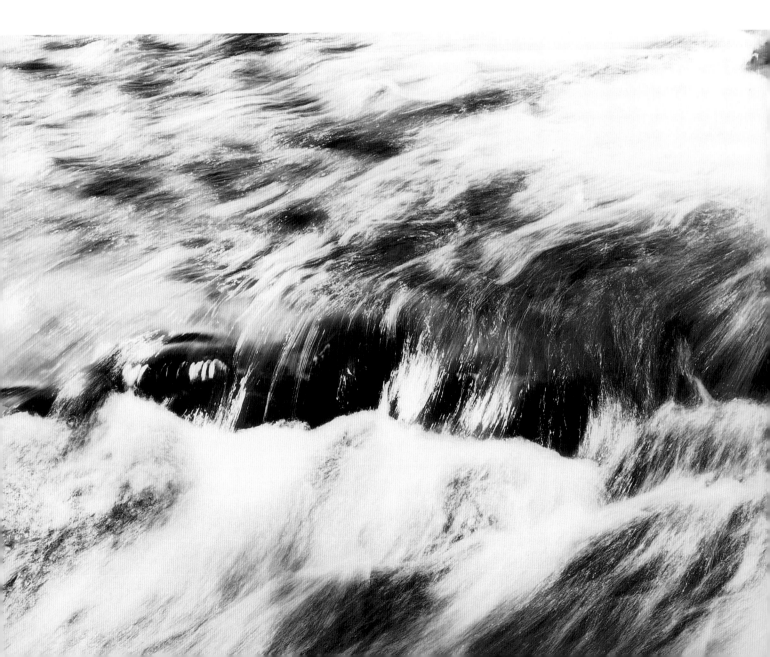

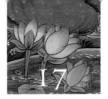

17

If beauty does lie in the heart, then Ayurveda (pro-

nounced Ay-yer-vay-dah) holds the key to unlocking

that inseparable mind-body-spirit beauty within. It

has been said that Vedic sciences are really a single

science with many windows. Vedic science, when

applied to health, could be called Ayurveda. In

Sanskrit, *ayu* means "life" and *veda* means "knowl-

edge." Ayurveda is a complete system of health for

the mind, body, and spirit. When the science is

applied to astrology, it is called *Jyotish*, and when applied to the body and the innate desire to cease feelings of separation, it is called yoga. Likewise, when it is applied to the home and environment, it is called *Vastu Shastra*.

Ayurveda says that there are five elements of nature: earth, water, fire, air, and space, which co-exist within each living organism. Of these five, three predominate. They are *Kapha,* or earth—a combination of water and earth; *Pitta,* or fire—a combination of fire and water; and *Vata,* or air. These elements are referred to as *doshas.* Doshas are the qualities that create imbalances in our bodies that tend to arise, and cause diseases when our health is not at its optimum level. This can be affected by a variety of things, including the environment, diet, stress, and general states of being. When addressed specifically, health and harmony can be restored. These doshas each have their own characteristics, some of which may align with parts of our own personalities or natures.

Ayurvedic doctors may diagnose individuals by observing these characteristics while talking with you or by having you fill out exten-sive questionnaires covering everything from your sleeping to your dietary habits, as they relate to your responsiveness to stress or anger. Then, they may read your pulse to determine your particular combination of the doshas. This is called the pulse diagnosis. Once they establish your dosha and learn any health concerns you may have, they might pre-scribe herbs for your condition that will help to regulate your body.

We each have varying degrees of all three doshas, but generally we are ruled by one or two dominant doshas at any given time. If you think of the elements in ascending order from the ground upward, they would read Kapha, Pitta, and Vata. Kapha, the combination of earth and water, would be the most grounded of the three doshas. Most of the characteris-tics of Kapha are qualities that come from being rooted in the earth. Those characteris-tics are intuition, stability, compassion, patience, and kindness. When out of balance, that energy can become lethargic, heavy, and sluggish. Kapha season is the spring, and is also considered the childhood within a life-time. The Kapha hours in the day are from six to ten in the morning and evening. Kaphas

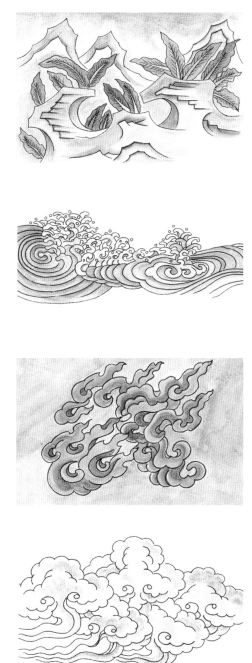

Earth—The earth has been worshiped as its own sacred god, or goddess—a living being with a soul. It is likely that all of its forms have or have had some meaning at one point or another. From volcanoes and mountains, to valleys and caves, the earth produces many symbolic features. Its products have inspired spiritual and mystical practices since the beginning of time (sacred tree worship, paganism, alchemy, and so forth), and many of its beautiful manifestations are still considered to hold sacred powers today.

Water—The magical properties of water are great. Another universal symbol for the soul, water possesses the power to cleanse, heal, and transform. Water provides transportation and sets boundaries here on earth, as well as within the spiritual realm. In Hinduism, rivers, for example, symbolize purification. In Christianity, baptism in water provides the ritualized "washing away" of one's sins. Islam places an important emphasis on water in its depictions of heavenly paradise. Water's personality is as diverse as its many different forms.

Fire—Fire has been revered as the source of light and the essence of divinity. It creates and destroys, and is associated with things both demonic and divine. It is used in many rituals in every religion and is often a symbol of the soul.

Air—Circulating throughout the body and universe, air carries the vital energy, *prana*. Air is the most intangible of the elements, yet it is necessary to animate all living creatures. Air represents the freedom connoted by such things as the sky, wind, flight, and breath.

tend to have strong, solid body types and have abundant dark hair. Kapha skin tends toward oiliness, especially in youth, but this will help to preserve the skin in adulthood.

Pitta, the combination of water and fire, would come next. Pitta characteristics are of a generally fiery nature and include passion, discipline, and leadership. When out of balance, Pittas are apt to short tempers and agitation. Pitta season is the summer and is reflected in a lifetime as middle age. Correspondingly, midday is Pitta's prime time. Physical attributes may be red hair and freckled skin, which may be normal or combination, and can also be prone to rashes and other skin conditions.

Vata, the combined elements of air and space, is the dosha most associated with spirit. Vata is the golden age in a lifetime, but is of the winter season. Vatas are creative, animated, and social creatures when balanced, but when not balanced, they have short attention spans and can be flighty. Their skin tends to be dry and their bone structure is usually petite.

But Ayurveda is more than an assessment of our outward characteristics and typical skin types. Much, much more. It is India's 5,000-year-old system of health and healing. And, unlike most of Western medicine, Ayurveda is also inclusively and especially attentive to the realities of the feminine body, mind, and emotional being. This traditional "life-science" addresses aspects of our world and ourselves that are not necessarily obvious physical factors.

There are so many elements, seen and unseen, that play a vital role in our inner and outer health. Life is full of relationships. We have relationships with ourselves, with other people, with nature, with society, and with our varied environments. We are constantly seeking and taking in everything from love and emotions to food and sounds. The flow between and amongst all of these has an impact on our health—mentally, spiritually, and physically. And all too often we desperately seek from outside sources the answers that are naturally hidden inside of us. Rather than trying to fix what's inside or fill those holes with the impermanencies that the world has to offer, Ayurveda strives to do just the opposite—to work inside out, joining our mental awareness to our physical body. By becoming an integrated being, we are thus more aptly integrated with nature.

Ayurveda also recognizes the complex symbiotic relationship between the awarenesses within our beings. Just as each of our organs and parts possesses its own awareness, our mind and spirit is equally aware. By this reality, each of our thoughts affects our organs and parts and, conversely, what affects our physical parts (like the injection of a chemical or a toxic release) in turn affects our mind. These principles of mind-body medicine go one step further in Ayurveda to include—perhaps the most important element in the equation—the soul. It is impossible to eliminate consciousness and the spirit in the assessment and promotion of one's health. Within each of us, and in the universe at large, there flows a vital energy called prana. This "life force" is the shakti (energy) of our beings. It can be invigorating or it can be unconstructive, depending on how we learn to circulate and balance it.

Ayurveda allows us to achieve the healthy balance between our minds, bodies, and spirits that we so often seek in vain. Once we are able to maintain this happy equilibrium, taking into account our doshas and the complexities of our relationships, we radiate with life and inspire the true beauty that flows from inner to outer.

Chakras

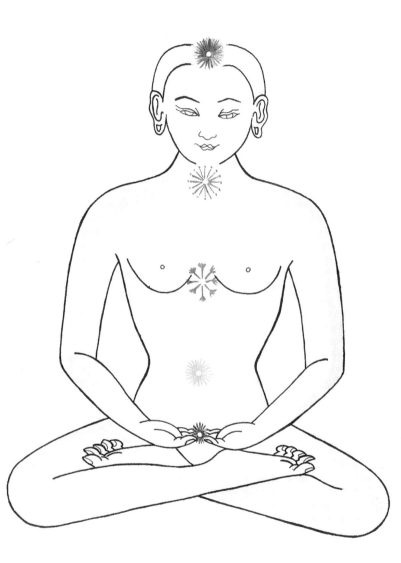

Fundamental to the practice of yoga, primarily Tantric and Hatha traditions, is the scientific belief of the East that alongside the physical body exists an etheric, or "subtle," body that has its own energy system. Within this system there are specific channels, called *nadi*, through which prana flows, enters, and leaves. There are three main channels—*ida, pingala,* and *susumna*—that all run along and around the spinal column, from the crown of the head to the base of the spine. At the points where these three channels intersect along the spinal column (typically seven) are concentrated centers of prana known as chakras. For most, the amount of prana that flows through the chakras is just enough to sustain our lives at a basic level. Through meditation and yoga, however, it is possible for the practitioner to harness that prana energy and carry it up through the chakras, unlocking and releasing spiritual and emotional energy. It is also along one of these nadi channels, at the lowest chakra, that the kundalini serpent is coiled, blocking the upward flow of prana.

Translated, *chakra* means "wheel." It is said that at the chakras, the prana that flows through the nadis forms bright, spinning wheels of light. In a yogi, the chakras exist as vibrant shining circles, as yoga allows the practitioner to experience them more fully through the awakening and encouraging of prana flow. A balanced flow of prana is directly connected to physical and emotional health, and it is possible to enhance the energy of certain chakras by focusing on them through yoga practice (Kundalini or otherwise). Visualizing the chakras, their colors, their locations, and chanting the associated mantra, is a great meditation tool, not to mention an instrument for experiencing higher spiritual states.

Each chakra has a distinct set of characteristics and is associated with a specific part of the body. In addition, the chakras all have their own mantra "seeds," or *bija*. The Hindu tradition typically depicts seven chakras and associates a deity (both male and female) to each, as well. In the tradition of Tibetan Buddhism, there are five. The chakras shown here are: *ajna, vishuddha, anahata, manipura,* and *swadhisthana.*

- Sahasrara, also referred to by Buddhists as the nirvana chakra, is the "thousand-petaled lotus," situated at the crown of the head. Technically, sahasrara is not really part of the chakra system, but is the place where the physical body is transcended. The thousand petals are white or golden and are associated with the seed mantra OM. Sahasrara is associated with the higher mind and union with the Absolute. In addition to Para-Brahman, this crown chakra is ruled by Siva, whose symbol is placed in the middle of the lotus.

- Ajna, also known as the "third eye." This chakra is located in the brain and externally depicted on the forehead, midway between the eyes. It is also called the "guru chakra" because it is said that it is through this point that the student receives telepathic communication from the teacher. It is associated with the sense of individuality and intuition and with the seed mantra OM. Its symbol is a bluish-gray, two-petaled lotus circumscribing a phallic symbol and downward-pointing triangle. The presiding deities are Parama-Shiva and Hakini, and ajna is also associated with the supreme element.

- Vishudda, "pure." Located at the throat, this chakra is represented as a sky-blue sixteen-petaled lotus whose symbol is the snowy-white elephant (strength). Vishudda chakra is associated with the element ether, the sense of hearing, the mouth, lungs, and skin, and the mantra *ham*. It is here at this center that the nectar of immortality is produced. The presiding deities are Ardhanarishvara and Shakini.

- Anahata translates to "unstruck." The anahata chakra is located at the heart and is therefore sometimes called the "heart lotus." It is represented by a blue or green lotus of twelve petals. It is at the heart that the transcendental sound, the vibration of the universe, is heard. This chakra is associated with the element air, the sense of touch, the heart, the lungs, and the mantra *yam*. It is also symbolized by a black antelope (speed) and is presided over by Isha and the goddess Kakini.

- Manipura means "jewel city." The manipura chakra is situated at the navel and is therefore related to the abdomen, back, spleen, stomach, and digestive system. It is represented by a yellow lotus with ten petals and is associated with the sense of sight, the element of fire, the mantra *ram*, the animal ram (fiery energy), and the feet. This chakra is presided over by Rudra and Lakini.

- Swadhisthana translates into "own base" and is located at the genitals. This chakra is associated with the hands, reproductive organs, the sense of taste, and the element water. The swadhisthana chakra holds the center for creativity and sexual energy and is depicted as an orange or crimson-colored six-petaled lotus. The crocodile (fertility) is associated with it, as is the mantra *vam*. Vishnu and Rakini are its presiding deities.

- Muladhara means "root support." This chakra is located at the perineum (between the anus and the genitals), which is also called *adhara*. This center is associated with the element earth, the sense of smell, and the legs. It is here that the kundalini is coiled. The muladhara chakra is represented by a deep red lotus with four petals and associated with the mantra *lam* and the elephant (strength).

Kabbalah

Perhaps to the newcomer, the tradition of yoga, and all of the associated sacred texts and symbology, seem quite "far out" or mystical, at first. But it certainly isn't the only esoteric system of spiritual philosophy to exist and still be practiced today by modern seekers searching for a personal path.

The Kabbalah, an elaborate system of arcane and practical wisdom, offers a spiritual path to awakening to students of the Hebrew tradition, though it has been and is often interpreted by Christians. The Kabbalah teaches a mystical philosophy, based on a system of symbols, numerology, and holy scriptures, meant to unlock the mysteries of God and creation.

There are even specific parallels that can be drawn between Kabbalistic teaching and yogic beliefs. For example, the Kabbalah, also an originally oral tradition, can be accessed through a diagram called the "sefiroth," or "tree of life." This diagram can be applied to virtually anything—from the human anatomy to the design of a house—just as a mandala can be made so widely applicable, as well. Within this mystical Jewish system, the center of the body is believed to be alive with knowledge. According to the Kabbalah, there are seven spheres of heavenly power located along central channels through the anatomy, much like the seven chakras within yoga.

Sarvangasana
(shoulder stand)

Sarvangasana is one of the most beneficial of all the asanas. Some say sirsasana is king of the asanas, and sarvangasana is the queen. Sarvangasana develops the feminine qualities of patience and emotional stability (again, as stated in *Yoga: A Gem for Women*). This asana strives for peace and bodily health. Sarvangasana affects the entire system. Like sirsasana, sarvangasana's inverted position uses gravity to pull the blood flow. But unlike sirsasana, the areas that most benefit from the increased circulation are the heart, chest area, and throat. This asana involves a firm chin-lock that directs a supply of blood to the thyroid and parathyroid glands, increasing their efficiency in function. This chin-lock also keeps the head in a firm position, which results in soothed nerves and the calming of the mind, and can even alleviate headaches and colds. As sarvangasana is soothing to the nervous system, this is a good pose to practice when one is feeling stressed, irritated, or fatigued. It is also a superior aid to digestion and elimination, urinary, and menstrual problems. Mentally, sarvangasana brings to the practitioner peace, strength, vigor, and vital longevity.

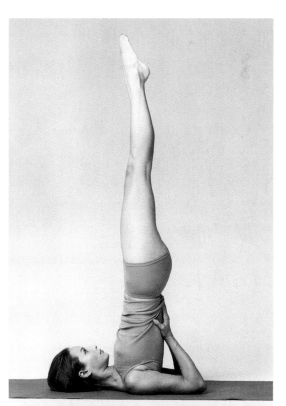

WHAT IS VASTU?

Creating a Sacred Space

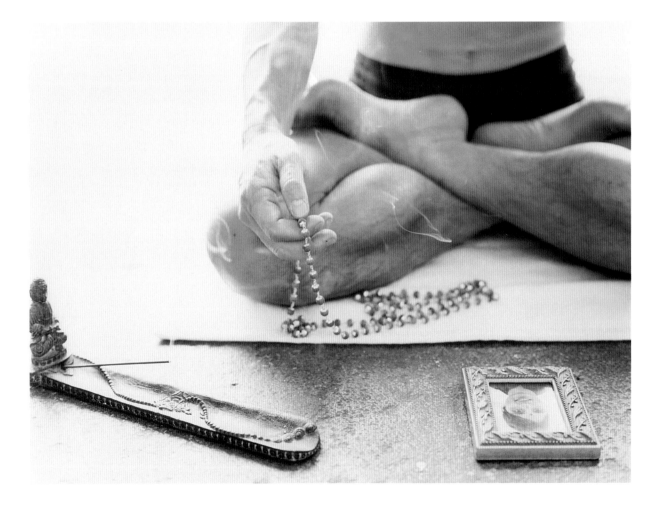

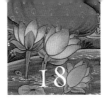

18

Sacred space is an integral part of living yogically. We can achieve temporary states of bliss in a yoga class or in meditation practice but, to have lasting results, it helps to also make changes within our homes and in our work environments. Modern life presents us with so many challenges, even if we do have a spiritual practice. We have taken on so many roles in our lives—daughter, sister, colleague, friend, mother, partner, and so on—we are often left feeling drained, empty, unequipped, or like a failure in any one area at a given point in the day, week, or month. We often feel that it's impossible to meet the needs of everyone around us, especially ourselves. There is no single answer here, only possibilities to solutions. Let us start with the home. This is the place where we begin and end most of our days. It should be a private sanctuary where we can retreat to when we feel overwhelmed.

In dreams, the home often represents the self, according to Carl Gustav Jung. The home can be seen as an extension or expression of the self, just as the walls of teenagers' bedrooms are often covered with things that are important to them. Posters, books, and photos turn each of these bedrooms into a refuge from the world; a place where they can be who they want to be. When we have such a space in which to reflect, we remember who we are and what we value. And in every home, no matter what size, there are places that can bring us happiness and offer us comfort and security. As with many things in life, it is important to remember that it is not always what is on the outside that is most important. We can apply

that philosophy to our spaces, as well. And a good way to start thinking about that space is through the science of *Vastu*.

Kathleen Cox, author of *Vastu Living: Creating a Home for the Soul* and *The Power of Vastu Living*, claims, "Vastu is an extension of yoga, meditation, ayurveda, the [musical form] raga and Indian classical dance—which are all about balance and perfect harmony. When you design your space so that it promotes inner peace, you're more likely to achieve your goals." Vastu treats a physical place or building, while yoga treats the body and spirit. Vastu, which is Sanskrit for "dwelling" or "site," uses architectural design to balance a structure so that it is aligned with the governing rhythms of the universe. This creates an environment that fosters health, happiness, and prosperity. I met with Kathleen, and she eloquently explained the following . . .

Vastu is forgiving. It accepts that we mortals are imperfect. Only God and the elements are perfect. Accordingly, Vastu shows us how to arrange our homes so that they acknowledge the body's imperfection. If you look at your body, it is asymmetrical—your hands and feet, your eyes and eyebrows. And the body is not the exception to the rule; most everything in nature is asymmetrical. Just examine a leaf on a plant. The Vastu guidelines for the placement of furnishings and the arrangement of décor honor asymmetry, not symmetry. And we discover through the practice of Vastu that we feel more comfortable sitting in a space that is arranged asymmetrically.

Vastu scholars believe that the home is a living organism, where the center of each room is considered the womb or navel, which is also the center of the human body. Since all creation begins here, the womb and navel are sacred. They should be protected from any weight and left uncovered so that creative energy can circulate, unhindered.

The northeast quadrant in Vastu also has a sacred dimension. The healthiest rays of the sun, which come with the dawn and continue into the early morning, flow into this quadrant. The first light of day is calming and a source of rejuvenation. Yogis try to face this direction when they meditate. In Vastu, the northeast quadrant of every space, even if we don't receive this light, should symbolically honor the restoring power of the early morning sun, which helps us turn inward.

According to Kathleen, this quadrant is ideal for a zone of tranquility, which draws our attention to this therapeutic part of a room. The zone can be small, but it should display something that connects to nature, such as a lovely flower or appealing terra-cotta sculpture, and a second object that relates powerfully to our personal life and fills us with love. When we feel overwhelmed by the demands of the day, we can focus on our zone of tranquility. Our personal display helps us empty our mind of unhealthy clutter and makes us mindful of our blessings. We reconnect to what really matters in our life.

Vastu also reminds us that when we open our eyes in the morning, the first thing we see in our bedroom should fill us with joy and present us with a positive greeting. So Vastu suggests that we place something on a wall or table (but always in our direct line of vision) that makes us feel good at the start of each day. Ultimately, Vastu helps us create a home that honors our extraordinary universe and celebrates the sacred nature of all existence, and that includes every one of us and every one who enters our home and our life.

Of course, like most things in yoga and in life, there is a history behind Vastu. Its history combines sacred geometry with modern physics and Hindu mythology with common sense. And, like its sister science, yoga, Vastu's history reaches back thousands of years.

Vastu is the Vedic science of architecture and interior design. The collected wisdom of the Hindu Vedas was put into writing at least 5,000 years ago. The Vedas are divided into four texts (Rig, Yajur, Sama, and Atharva) and describe the sacred laws of nature, the creative energies of the universe, and the mythology of the Vedic gods and goddesses. Ayurveda, the world's first science of health, was first expounded in the Vedas. Yoga, a sister science of Ayurveda, was also first articulated here, as was Vastu.

The Vedas teach us that we stay in good health when we live in a state of harmony with nature. Through the practice of the Vedic disciplines, we can move closer toward the awakening of the true self. Both Ayurveda and Vastu are concerned with maintaining good health. But while Ayurveda focuses on the body, Vastu focuses on the environments that surround the body. The Vedic philosophy states that everything in the universe is interconnected and interdependent, and that all creation observes a series of natural laws that govern the workings of the universe. Through the practice of Vastu, we try to orient our home so that it honors these theories. And by creating order and balance in our home, we mirror the order and balance that exists in the universe.

Vastu is Sanskrit for "dwelling" or "site." Vastu, like Ayurveda, is based on the Vedic theory of the creation of the universe. A popular Hindu myth tells of this moment in time. Eons ago, Brahman, who Hindus believe is the unseen yet powerful force behind all creation, assumed the form of Brahma, the god of creation. Brahma then re-created the five basic elements that existed within his own form to create the universe and all existence.

Lord Brahma created each of the elements,

one by one—from simple to complex, from light to heavy. First, Brahma created space (or ether); then Brahma created air, which can't exist without space; next came fire, which can't exist without space and air; next came water; and finally, earth.

Vastu assigns a specific area in every space to each one of the five basic elements. By paying attention to these locations when we design and organize our home, we honor these elements, which are at the heart of all creation. They exist within the human body, they exist in all of nature, they exist in every single thing in the Cosmos. Their presence within all creation helps us understand why everything is interconnected and interdependent. Everything is created by the same sacred source and has its role to play in the grand plan and deserves our respect.

The wisdom in this theory is apparent when we think about the presence of the five basic elements in our own body. These elements govern all the bodily functions that keep us alive. At the time of conception, we occupy space and require space in which to grow. Our breath draws in air and moves around the oxy-gen that is vital for our survival. Our digestive fire burns the calories that give us our energy. Nearly two thirds of our body is made up of water; without water, we could not survive. And where is earth? The properties of earth are in the minerals, from calcium to zinc, that keep our structure healthy.

To practice Vastu, we pay attention to a spiritual grid that is called the *vastu purusha mandala*. Most Eastern religions use mandalas, which are often symbolic depictions of the universe, as a point of focus in meditation. Typically, mandalas help us concentrate, turn inward, and move along the path to enlightenment. The vastu purusha mandala serves a similar purpose; it helps us succeed in our practice of Vastu. The two Sanskrit words, Vastu (dwelling or land) and purusha (unseen energy or spirit that lies within) combine together to mean the cosmic spirit of the dwelling or land. In Hinduism, there are many myths that explain the origin and importance of vastu purusha.

One story about the spirit Vastu Purusha recounts the existence, once upon a time, of an evil force, unnamed and without form, that extended across the firmament and threatened to destroy the universe. Heavenly deities became so alarmed that they begged Brahma to put an end to this destructive force. Brahma ordered the guardian deities of the eight directions to grab hold of this evil force and pull it down to earth. Then Brahma turned it into a spirit whose face was pressed into the ground.

Brahma sat with all his weight upon the spirit's navel and instructed the other deities to help hold down the creature so that it could never escape. The spirit was repentant, and out of compassion, Brahma gave it the name of Vastu Purusha—or the cosmic spirit of the land. Brahma also decided that Vastu Purusha had to be worshiped at the start of every construction. This would ensure the protection of the inhabitants of the new structure. Failure to appease him would lead to misfortune. When we appease Vastu Purusha, we are really honoring the Vastu guidelines and the principles that govern the universe. We create harmony and balance in our home and show respect for all creation.

The vastu purusha mandala shows the cosmic spirit inside a square mandala with his head in the east but bowed toward the northeast out of respect for this quadrant, which is also called the gateway to the gods. Vastu Purusha has one hand reaching into the northeast corner and the other reaching into the southeast corner. One foot is firmly placed in the northwest corner and the other is firmly placed in the southwest corner.

Four of the guardian deities, each one connected to a basic element, occupy these midpoint directions. Isa and the element of water are assigned to the northeast; Agni and the element of fire are assigned to the southeast; Pitri and the element of earth are assigned to the southwest; and Vayu and the element of air are assigned to the northwest. Brahma and the fifth element of space (ether) reign in the center. We can think of the guardian deities as restraining the hands and feet of Vastu Purusha; while Brahma, the lord of creation, is holding down the spirit's navel, which plays such a vital role in creation.

The Vedic theory that claims there is nothing random in the universe holds true in Vastu. There is nothing random about the placement of the guardian deities and the five basic elements on the vastu purusha mandala and within our home. The rhythms at work in the universe—the cycles that play out day after day as the earth travels around the sun—govern their placement. And if we organize our home so that we can maintain a state of harmony with these all-important rhythms, our home can increase our well-being and contribute to our good health.

The element of water and its deity, Isa (who later became known as Shiva, who is considered the *Mahadeva* or Great God and the god of yogis), reside in the northeast. The northeast receives the healthiest rays of the sun, which come as the sun rises slowly in the east, which some believe is the primary direction. The magnetic pull of the earth comes from the north. The midpoint between these two directions, which is the northeast, is called the gateway to the gods and is considered the source of positive cosmic energy or *prana*, the breath of life. Prana enters the northeast quadrant and travels in a wide arc to the southwest quadrant.

Vastu has assigned the element of water to the northeast because water is a receptacle that can collect and retain the cosmic energy. This potent gateway to the gods is also a source of calm and tranquility, two characteristics that we also connect with water. The northeast is the perfect location for a pond, swimming pool, or simply an open expanse that allows the early sun and healthy energy to flow freely into the property. In the home, water also belongs in the northeast quadrant. We should also try to keep our lightweight and delicate furnishings in this part of the room so that the cosmic energy can travel unobstructed into the southwest. The northeast, with its soothing properties, is an excellent location for a meditation room or study. Zones of tranquility, which help us calm down and reduce our stress, also belong in this quadrant.

The deity Agni, the Vedic god of fire, governs the southeast corner of the mandala along with the element of fire. Once again, the movement of the sun, which is directly overhead when it reaches this quadrant, determines their location. "Agni, called the light of knowledge, also represents the awakening of the soul," says Cox. This explains the presence of fire in most Hindu ceremonies. Fire purifies and, through the act of cremation, liberates the immortal soul from the perishable body.

In today's context, fire includes electricity and heating elements. So in the Vastu home, we try to keep electrical equipment and sources of heat in the southeast quadrant. The preferred location for the kitchen is also the southeast, where it can honor the role of the sun and fire in the creation of our body's nourishment. Plant life can't thrive without sunlight, so, directly or indirectly, all our food is dependent on the presence of the sun. Fire also demands our respect. It can burn us and do us harm; while its absence can bring about our demise.

Lord Pitri, who is the god of ancestors, rules over the southwest quadrant and the element of earth. Earth is heavy, dense, and strong. Earth also represents the final state of our existence. To dust, we all return. The element's connection with the lord of ancestors reinforces the quality of strength that is a physical property of earth. The wisdom left behind by the departed empowers each future generation. The world is enriched by what is left behind.

In Vastu, the placement of the element of earth in the southwest serves two important functions. The sun, moving across the south into the southwest, is unhealthy for us; we want to block out its harmful rays. We also want to keep the beneficial cosmic energy inside our home or property. So we mirror the properties of earth in our practice of Vastu. In the southwest of the property, we try to create density, heaviness, and height with a barrier of trees, a rock garden, or any thick growth. Inside the home, we try to place our tall and heavyweight furnishings in the southwest, where they can keep out the harmful sun and keep in the beneficial energies or pranic flow.

Vayu, the Vedic god of winds, rules in the northwest quadrant. His location connects to weather patterns in the Northern Hemisphere. The northwester represents the most volatile wind, so this quadrant is well-suited to Vayu and his element of air. Air, which is vital to all creation, symbolizes movement, which is a property of the wind. The wind is always on the go and definitely fickle. It can quickly change direction. In Vastu, this quadrant mirrors the properties of the wind. It is the ideal location for a guest

creating a home for the soul . . .

NORTHWEST	NORTH	NORTHEAST
Guest bedroom,	*Bedroom, library,*	*Meditation room*
dining room,	*dining room*	*or shrine*
TV, bathroom		
WEST	SACRED CENTER	EAST
Bedroom,	*Atrium,*	*Studio, bedroom,*
living room,	*spacious living room*	*dining room*
dining room, library		
SOUTHWEST	SOUTH	SOUTHEAST
Living room, master	*Bathroom or*	*Kitchen or*
bedroom, storage	*bedroom*	*electronics*

"The square is usually divided into nine subsections, with each section representing one of the eight cardinal directions/gods who sat on Purusha, with Brahma in the ninth and center box."

bedroom, where people come and go. It's a perfect spot for a TV if you watch hour after hour. The properties associated with the northwest will make you restless and therefore you will move on.

Lastly, Brahma, the Creator, governs the element of space, which is at the center of the vastu purusha mandala. This sacred area is called the *Brahmasthana* (or the place of Brahma), which is the source of creative energy. This energy, which circulates through every space, creates positive vibrations that reinvigorate us and inspire us. Since we want to receive this important energy, we try not to cover the sacred center of any Vastu space.

In Vastu, the remaining four guardian deities, who remind us of the importance of duality, govern the cardinal directions of north, south, east, and west. The east speaks of light and clarity, the west of darkness and the unknown. We can't appreciate the light without experiencing the dark. The north represents health, wealth, and indulgence; while the south represents duty, obligation, and death. If we overindulge or neglect our health, we suffer the consequences. So these four deities and the cardinal directions remind us to live in a state of balance—emotionally, physically, and mentally.

Having read about the role of the elements and the important deities, we can understand the chart that shows the recommended placement of the rooms that are apt to exist in a home. The center square belongs to Lord Brahma, who is surrounded by the eight squares occupied by the eight guardian deities who either represent an important element or an aspect of a duality—properties that reflect the principles that govern the universal world or the world of ethical behavior.

Few people can create a perfect sacred space. Many of us cannot change the location of our rooms to match the grid. But we can always shift around some furniture inside a room or modify our décor so that it respects nature and our own true self. The Vedas accept imperfection, so in Vastu, we strive to do our best. We pay attention to the power of our environment and the needs of our dosha. If we just do this, we can create our own personal sacred space.

Halasana
(plough pose)

In Sanskrit, *hala* means "plough." From a lying position, the feet are brought over the head toward the ground, resulting in a posture that resembles a plough.

With benefits similar to those of sarvangasana, this posture is known to calm the brain. It provides an extra supply of blood to the spine while stretching it, and is therefore therapeutic for back pain. Halasana helps relieve the symptoms of menopause, stretches the shoulders, stimulates the abdominal organs and the thyroid gland, and is a good reliever of stress and fatigue. In this posture, the interlocking and stretching of the hands and fingers helps to relieve hand cramps and can be beneficial for arthritis. One yogi suggests reflecting on "ploughing" our own lives and minds as we relax in this posture—to "weed out" that which is not healthy for ourselves, and to begin to sow seeds of understanding and growth.

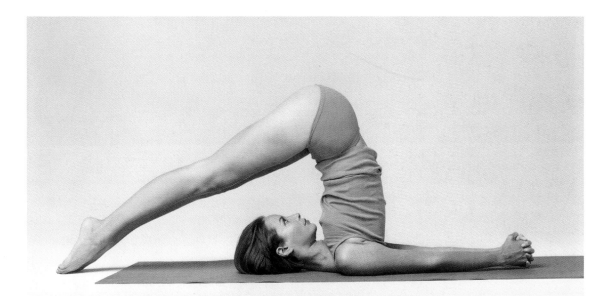

METAMORPHOSIS

"In the sky there is no East or West.
We make these distinctions in the mind, then believe them to be true."
—RUDOLPH WURLITZER IN *HARD TRAVEL TO SACRED PLACES*

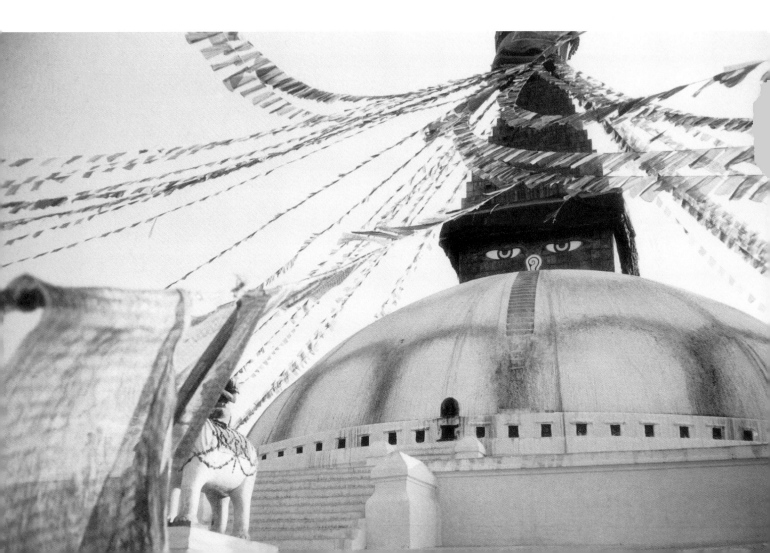

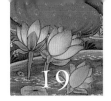

19

Upon graduation from school, I had been excitedly

planning a long trip to Africa, to climb Mt.

Kilimanjaro in Tanzania and travel around for a while

as a present to myself. I didn't want to rush into any

life-making decisions just yet. I needed time to

breathe and to pause between life's events. I was in

the midst of a major transition in my life, perhaps

the biggest yet, and I wanted to savor it.

A friend of mine had started an organization to save

the rain forest in the eastern arc of Africa, in Tanzania. For a few years already, I had been helping to raise funds to promote consciousness about the region through various efforts, and had wanted to visit the area to see what had been accomplished in terms of reforestation and education. I find that one of the great challenges of beginning and sustaining endeavors outside of our local communities, especially on a global scale, is to educate ourselves and take responsibility for how our actions may affect others; just as the actions of others, anyplace in the world, may affect ours. Rain forest preservation is so important and necessary in the ecological balance of our planet, and I wanted to be involved in that.

I had been to that part of Africa on location for a shoot many years before, and had always hoped to return. In fact, I had promised myself that if I were ever to return, it would be to come back to climb Mt. Kilimanjaro, the highest peak in Africa (19,710 feet). So, a few weeks after graduation, I set out for my journey. I felt like I was on top of the world. As though I could do almost anything, be any-

one. I knew that this journey would bring me closer to that end, whatever it may be.

The first time I saw Mt. Kilimanjaro was during that first visit to Tanzania. I was on my way to neighboring Kenya, where my parents were also traveling, when I flew over the impressive peak (the mountain sits close to the borders of both countries). It took my breath away. Now, years later, after I had thrown myself deep into my studies immediately after my dad died, and had graduated with honors—how I wished he'd been there to congratulate me—I was still seeking out his spirit, following in his footsteps. We had shared a love of travel and adventure, and I think that I longed to return to Africa, his dream destination, to reunite with his memory.

One of my father's final trips was to Africa in 1995, not long before he died. I had sent him on a lifelong dream hunting expedition: to seek out a Cape buffalo. I had been a longtime animal rights proponent, and though I was completely opposed to my father's boyhood ritual of hunting wild game, I assisted his adventure anyway. He had already traveled near and far for bear, pheasant, wild duck, elk, and deer for the whole of my life. I remember endless trips on which my sisters and I would accompany him to remote locations and sit and wait quietly while he was stalking some poor creature. It was such a part of him, like his smoking, that it was impossible to convince him that there was anything at all wrong with it. I think that what he most enjoyed about it was the silence. He was a quiet man, and being outdoors was a mission of sorts. Whether or nor I understood or agreed with hunting, it somehow allowed him to commune with nature and with his deceased father, who had passed the sport along when my father was a boy. What he didn't realize was that the journey was more important than the goal. Perhaps he could have achieved the same feeling without causing harm to another living creature.

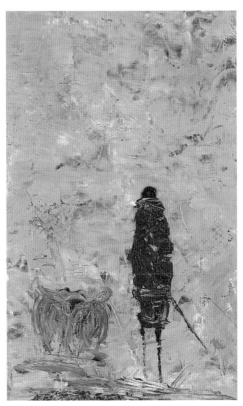

Besides his quiet disposition and ironic relationship with nature, my father was Hemingway-esque in many other ways, as well. He was tall and quintessentially American, both in principles and physique. We had shared a favorite Hemingway short story entitled "The Snows of Kilimanjaro." It is a tale about a man with a talent who marries into a higher social stratum, becomes spoiled, loses his drive, and, eventually, dies because of it. As a person completely out of his element, he loses himself in the vortex that he has created for himself. The story is a metaphor about the dangers of delusion. In real life, it is a tragedy to witness this all-too-common scenario happening to someone you know, and an even greater challenge to avoid it yourself. Reality checks are important for us all, and my own return to Africa was an important crossroad.

One of my life teachers often reminds me that we are what we seek.

We arrived in Arusha in late June. I had caught a chest infection a few days before we began our climb in the rain forest on the way from Dar es Salaam. From what I'd read on the way over, I knew that altitude could play a dangerous role in such an infection, and I willed my way back to health almost overnight. We started the trek at 7,000 feet on a misty midafternoon. We were bent on learning some of the national language, so our amazing local guides kept us engaged by attempting to teach us Swahili as we wound our way up to the first camp.

Each day, the temperatures grew colder as the altitude increased. We traversed through seven different zones of nature as we scaled up one of the many faces of this awesome mountain. On the second night, it began to snow when we set up our camp. There's a lot of time to think when you are summoned to your tent at five in the afternoon because the fire cannot sustain itself amidst the flurries. Needless to say, I started to get to know myself pretty well.

Late that same night, I was forced to crawl out of my small but warm abode, a two-person tent, in search of our makeshift john at the edge of camp. The sky had cleared and was ultra-bright, and for the first time I could see the tabletop peak of the mountain we were climbing. It was a strange but familiar sensation to feel a part of something so great that was not wholly visible to me. Up until that moment, all I could do was to try to imagine what beauty might lie ahead, when I was unexpectedly given this glimpse of what awaited us. What I then saw was almost clichéd—like in the movies when the main character, during a long and perilous journey, awakens to find the clouds parting like stage curtains, revealing the new horizon. Yes, it was dramatic. But quietly so, subtly. I was truly awed. Somewhere, off in the distance, I could hear Hemingway: *"Then they began to climb and they were going to the East it seemed, and then it darkened and they were in a storm, the rain so thick it seemed like flying through a waterfall, and then they were out and Compie turned his head and grinned and pointed and there, ahead, all he could see, as wide as all the world, great, high, and unbelievably white in the sun, was the square top of*

Kilimanjaro. And then he knew that there was where he was going."

The next day, when we reached close to 15,000 feet, I experienced my only side effect from the altitude, which was a funny butterfly sensation in my belly. Fortunately, that passed after a day or so. It got colder and colder as we climbed, but my feet were the only thing on my body that felt it. I practiced a walking technique the guides taught us that helped a lot as the air thinned and the terrain steepened. I forced myself to breathe in time to each step so that it naturally evolved into a sort of walking meditation—pranayama on the slopes of Mt. Kilimanjaro.

When we were all spread out a bit, each in our own world of thought or non-thought, it was easy to lose myself in my rhythmic breathing. I found myself "sensing" the journey, no longer merely walking it. I sometimes felt that I was my father as I walked along, strong and proud. At other moments, I could as easily have been walking amongst the intricate lines of a labyrinth. Looking down from where we were to where we had come from, there was a

vast expanse of whiteness, a blank canvas. But where we were going was pulling us forward.

We gravitated upward and sang our progress in Swahili through motivational hymns. We chanted:

Tembea na Yesu Amen
Haleluya Amen
Ukiwa Mlimani- Amen
Ukiwa Kazini
Tembea ne Yesu
Amen Haleluya Amen

Walk with me, Jesus
On the mountain
Everywhere
Walk with me, Jesus

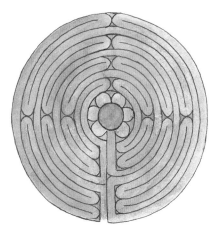

The eve before we were supposed to reach the peak, one of our friends was taken down the mountain in an emergency evacuation because he was suffering so badly from altitude sickness. Half the camp went with him to set up a safe place for him to re-acclimate, while the rest of us spent a somber evening together worrying about his condition and apprehending our final ascent of the next morning. We woke at 4:30 A.M. I slept terribly, but had dreamt of my father shortly before waking. In the dream, he was in his very sick stage, though still alive. He wanted to give me something for my journey—a small book containing photographs of me taken at different stages of my life. I took the album from him, and then my younger sister drove me to the San Francisco airport, as she had done so many times when Dad was sick and I came home to visit. This was all I could remember, but it stayed with me throughout the rest of that final climb upward.

I led the group, taking slow, measured steps, till I reached the end of the rocky trail. All I could see was solid whiteness against a backdrop of white clouds. I could see faint feet tracks beneath my own, hardened in the ice on a seemingly little-traveled pathway leading to the summit. I followed it, shortening the distance between me and the tiny figures ahead at the summit. It was remarkably peaceful, just the soft crunching of the snow beneath my steps. When I was near enough to hear other people, I stopped to turn around one last time toward my group and the journey behind us. I turned again and looked at my feet, where a small butterfly lay dead on the path. I wondered how this tiny thing could have gotten all the way up here. I thought of picking it up and taking it with me, but decided against it and kept walking.

Despite the cold, I was elated at long last to have reached the top. At the summit stood a sign that said: "Uhuru Summit, the highest peak in Africa," with colorful Tara prayer flags streaming in the wind. These flags typically flutter around the Himalayan Mountain passes around Mt. Everest, as well as in Lhasa, the capital of Tibet. They were decorated by using wood blocks hand-carved with images and prayers to Lung-ta, the mythical wind horse who carries prayers for good fortune to the universe, and to Tara, the goddess who grants all wishes. Looking out over the land below, I learned that *Uhuru* means liberation, and is the purpose of most pilgrimages. This journey had liberated me from the life I had known, and now I was ready to begin again.

Pindasana (embryo pose) in Sarvangasana

This asana resembles, quite beautifully, an embryo. When practiced in sarvangasana, the benefits are focused on toning the abdominal organs and aiding digestion. The inverted position of the body in this posture helps, again, in the flow and purification of the blood. The increased blood circulation around the endocrine glands, especially the thyroid and parathyroid, is an important benefit.

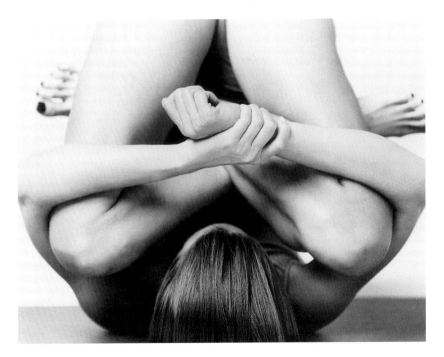

Uttana Padasana
(raised-feet posture)

Uttana padasana tones the neck and strengthens the back. *Uttana* means "stretched out on the back with the face up." *Pada* means "leg." Both the feet and the arms are raised in this posture, and the back is raised off the floor and arched. This asana fully opens the chest region and encourages suppleness in the spine. By increasing blood supply to the area, uttana padasana also balances thyroid activity.

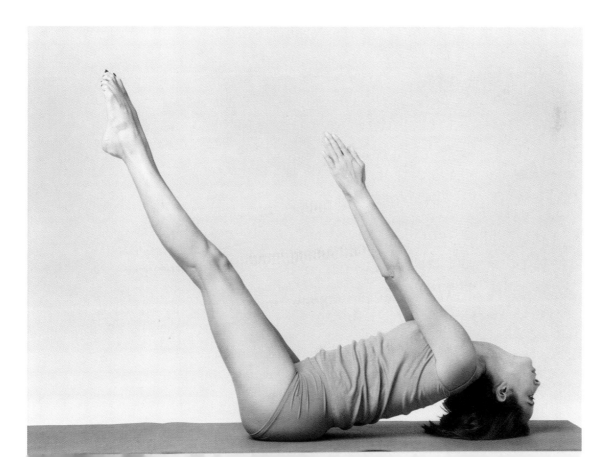

PILGRIMAGE

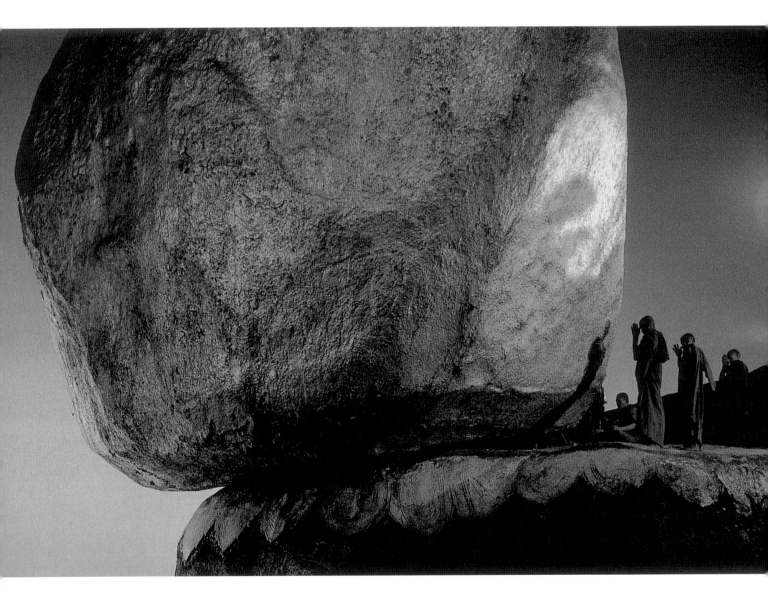

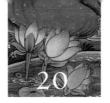

20

So much of our lives is spent traveling (these days).

We travel every day, to and from our homes, work,

the supermarket, the movies, in vehicles, in airplanes,

and even from our couches and through the pages of

our favorite books. But for as much traveling as we

do or perceive that we do, sometimes it simply is not

enough. We long for something more, something

meaningful. We long for the journey. For some of us,

this search takes us down both secular and spiritual

paths, and often to a crossroads. What begins as a trip, seeking whatever it is that is meaningful for the journeyer, turns into a spiritually reviving quest.

In some cultures, pilgrimage is a religious commandment. For many of us, though, it ranges from the all-inclusive evangelical tour to the pursuit of self-realization and spiritual enlightenment. Pilgrims have long traversed this earth, and the notion of such a journey is nothing surprising or new. During the Middle Ages, Christians traveled extensive distances to Canterbury and Santiago de Compostela, and even now some plan their vacation time around Jerusalem and Lourdes. Buddhists and Hindus have long sought the sacred waters of the Ganges River, and Muslims, at least once in their lifetime, are required to embark on the *hajj* to Mecca.

Today, modern pilgrims still carry on these traditions and are even creating new ones. I know American veterans who have made pilgrimages to Normandy, France, and family members of death camp victims who return to Europe seeking the spirits of those persecuted. Even Annie Dillard, in *Pilgrim at Tinker Creek*, found spiritual travel in her own backyard. For Hindus and other spiritual travelers, many of whom are yogis, one of the greatest sacred journeys is the *Kumbh Mela*.

The Kumbh Mela

My profession has taken me all over the globe, but India was a place I had saved for myself. I believed that I had to spend a significant amount of time there if I ever got the chance to go; if I ever got the opportunity as opposed to the usual few days that I am normally limited to, which would not be sufficient. Throughout recent years, my interest in India deepened through my studies, as well as through my yoga practice as it became a more integral part of my life. As I became more committed to my sadhana and yogic practices, which were developing into a lifestyle, I decided that I was ready to go.

I applied toward the end of my senior year of college to stay at an ashram in Ganeshpuri. I wrote a letter asking to stay for the month of

October—I had heard from friends that it was a good month, weatherwise—and waited to hear back. When I learned that I had not been accepted due to a lack of space, I decided to keep my plan but travel around India, rather than stay in one place. That summer I traveled a lot, as some do when they graduate from college, even if they are thirty years old. I spent a month in Africa, where I climbed Mt. Kilimanjaro and safaried in the Masai Mara, before heading home by way of Florence, where I stopped to spend a week at a yoga retreat hosted by two of my yoga teachers from New York, Sharon Gannon and David Life of the Jivamukti Yoga Center. It was here that I met and made friends with my future guides to India, Shyam and Tulsi.

Shyam and Tulsi live half the year in India and the other half in Woodstock, New York. He is a sharp and exuberant American and self-described pundit, and she is a regal Canadian who first met Shyam in India, where they later married, the year prior to our introduction. When they heard me speak of my plans of coming to India that fall, they kindly volunteered to show me around, and we began to plan an itinerary almost immediately. There is an expres-sion in India that says the guest is God, so Hindus are often incredibly gracious hosts.

We decided to meet in Delhi, and then travel into the Himalayas to Badrinath, and then on through the northern state of U.P. (Uttar Pradesh). During my final semester of school, I had taken a course called "Spiritual Journeys and Temporal Geographies," which ignited a fascination in pilgrimage. In this class, we explored the meanings of pilgrimage in the Abrahamic religions (Judaism, Christianity, and Islam) in particular, but also within various other cultures. We explored the common elements, such as the secular and spiritual dimensions, that transcend culture and religion. I had come to see all travel as an opportunity for transformation, and began to seek out occasions to experience true pilgrimage.

India is, and has been, considered a holy land to millions for centuries because it is filled with sacred sites. Out of these sites, we chose to visit Badrinath, one of the most important pilgrimage sites in all of India, located up high in the Himalayas, near the border of Tibet. Shyam and Tulsi are practicing Hindus, and are deeply devoted Vaishnavites (wor-

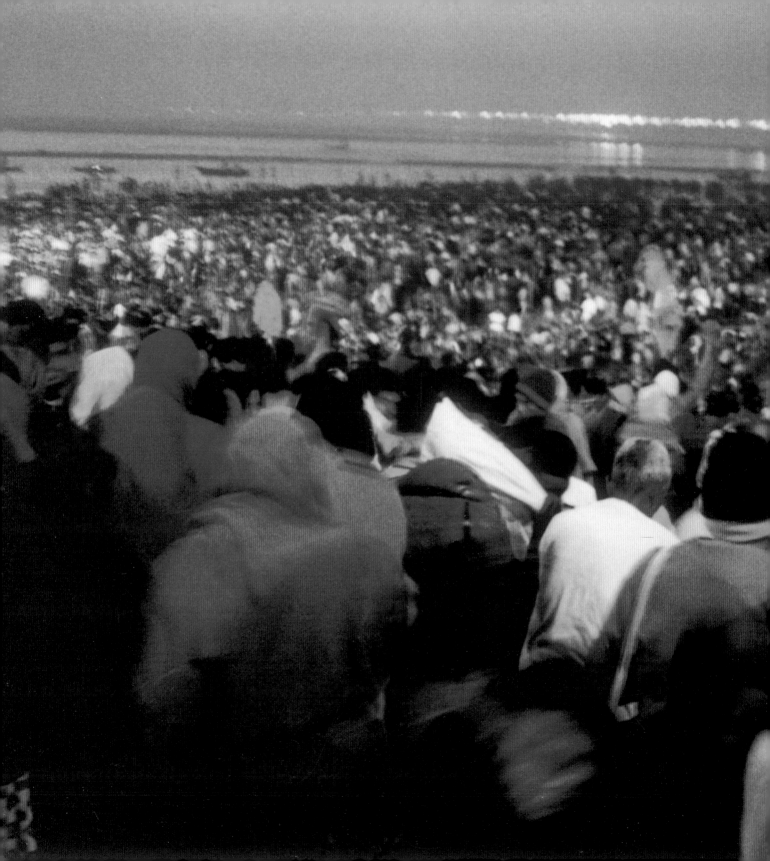

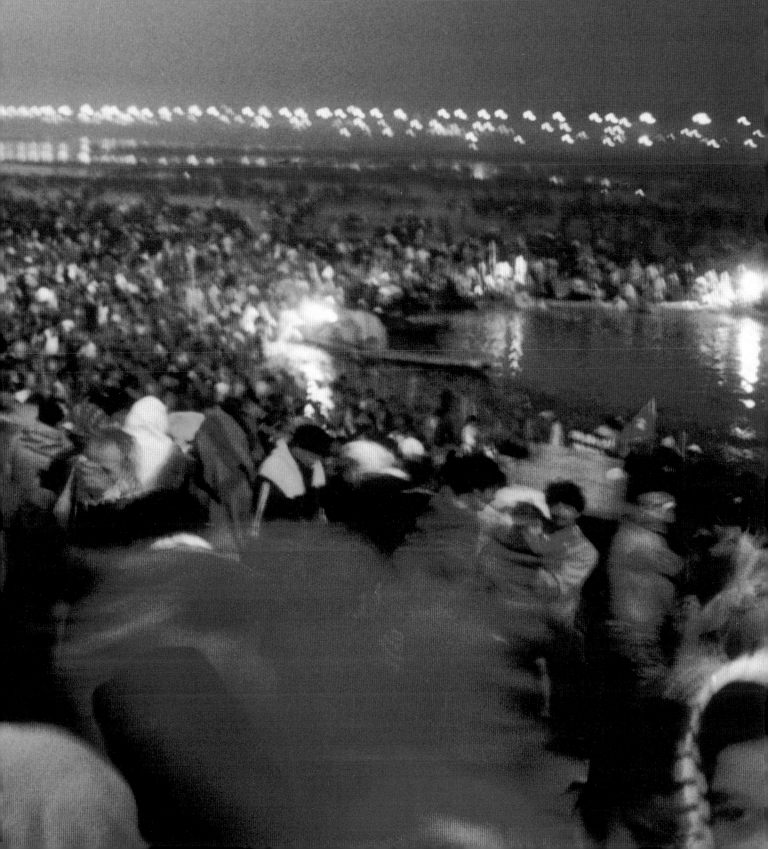

shipers of Vishnu) and practitioners of Bhakti (devotional) Yoga. They live in the state of U.P. because it is where Lord Krishna is said to have lived and played. I knew a bit about Bhakti Yoga from my studies of Hinduism, but I was delighted to journey to India for the first time with such devout practitioners, which promised to deepen my understanding, thus enriching my experience.

We decided to study the Bhagavad Gita along the way, and we compared translations of several texts during daily satsangs (a gathering centered around a spiritual leader or teaching), as Shyam would explain the translations in depth. When we reached Badrinath, I learned how to respectfully behave when inside a temple by following Tulsi's every move. She had taken me to purchase a few saris when we arrived in Delhi and showed me how to wrap myself appropriately, honoring the culture and the deities within the temples themselves. They taught me the proper etiquette for everything from eating from my right hand to drinking from a bottle without touching it to my mouth. I also learned how to bathe publicly.

Our first stop on the road to our destination was in Haridwar, located on the Ganges. Within an hour of reaching the guesthouse where we'd spend our first night, we changed out of our clothes, wrapped ourselves, and went down to the water's edge for a bath in the swiftly moving sacred source. There were support bars alongside that I held on to while dipping thrice below the sun-splashed surface, as instructed. The feeling was invigorating. For a pilgrim, one bath alone in the sacred rivers of the Ganges is believed to be sufficient to cleanse the soul. I was told that if my journey were to stop right there, I could return to the States having made a legitimate pilgrimage.

For many Western yogis, there is a sense that journeying to India itself is a necessary pilgrimage and, within the country, there are countless opportunities to contemplate God. India is a microcosm, within which ordinary experiences seem heightened and magnified. Issues that need facing at home are sure to surface in one's consciousness while traveling here. Accepting the worldly realm as a wakeful dream is one of the goals that modern yogis aspire to.

As practitioners, we are all faced with the challenge of how to remain yogic in our daily lives.

There is an illusion that here, in India, this would be easier somehow, but in truth, you realize that the challenge is also relative. People appear to be working so hard everywhere you look, but there is still time to visit the temple daily, at least once, to make an offering. In India, everything seems interwoven—faith, family, and work are all one—and each faithful act can lead to Brahman (the transcendental Reality). In the East, everything is regarded as dharma, so all is accepted. Yoga is everywhere. For instance, rivers are worshiped as goddesses, and the confluences of some of those rivers are deemed especially sacred.

However, if we choose a dharmic path, our sadhana (personal path) will flourish no matter where we are. This was my realization when I returned from that first pilgrimage, as it was my incentive to return earlier the next year to experience the ultimate pilgrimage, the *Maha Kumbh Mela*. While there, I had made a commitment to myself to make at least one pilgrimage annually. I knew that the commitment itself would be as important as the journey.

Before I arrived, for the second time, in India in January 2001, all I knew about the Maha Kumbh Mela was that it is a spiritual celebration that occurs every twelve years in four locations to commemorate one of the many Hindu creation myths. Though the legend varies a bit from individual to individual, it is essentially an epic tale of the victory of gods over demons over the *kumbh* (pot) of immortality after Lord Vishnu promises to them the nectar inside if they churn an ocean of milk. When the kumbh finally appears, the demons try to steal it from Jayant, the god who holds it. The myth purports that when this battle was going on, several drops of the nectar contained in the pot spilled onto the earth in four locations—Haridwar, Ujjain, Nasik, and Allahabad, where Jayant stopped every third day to rest. Allahabad is considered the most sacred because of its auspicious location at the convergence of the Yamuna and Ganges rivers.

As my departure date grew nearer, and coverage of the opening bathing day with all the Naga holy men and sadhus graced the front page of *The New York Times*, my ignorance, and much of the world's, began to dissipate. I learned that there were approximately twenty to forty million other pilgrims expected to attend this holy site during the forty-day festival.

Then, just hours before boarding my flight, news that a monumental earthquake had struck the Gujarat region of India the previous morning reached the international airwaves. When I arrived, the headlines read loud and clear that this was a catastrophe far worse than the rest of the world was imagining. Each day the rising death tolls were printed alongside the Kumbh coverage of daily accounts of the traffic there. Suddenly the purpose of the pilgrimage, as well as the dharma, became crystal clear to me. We must accept these tragedies and come together in light of them. Sad events present the opportunity to commune with ourselves and with others. If we were to look at all strife as a blessing, it is no wonder that India and the East offer this wealth of spirituality, for their history has left a legacy of it.

Though the Kumbh reports mimicked the media sensationalism of the West, highlighting only the numbers, eccentrics, and famous visitors (including Sonia Gandhi and the Dalai Lama), when we arrived at the *sangam*, where the two rivers merge, and the fairground itself, I was both surprised and relieved that it was the ordinary people who were the real heart of this gathering. There

were day-trippers and *Kalpvasis*, those who stay the duration of forty days. There were middle-class and upper-middle-class families, as well as the very rich and very impoverished. It was a humbling community.

When we arrived on the eve of one of the final bathing days, it was like an exodus, with the majority of vehicles heading out in the opposite direction. Inside the Mela grounds, which had been erected and were being maintained by the Indian government, chaos abounded. The air was thick with dust, smoke, and blaring noise from rivaling loudspeakers in every direction. Once we found our camp and tent we had reserved through friends who had been staying there earlier in the week, we ventured outside to familiarize ourselves with our fellow pilgrims. Like Manhattan, where I live, Allahabad is a city that never sleeps, and the commonalities don't stop there. You could see the spectrum of humanity that coexists around the world each and every day. When traveling, I am always catching myself making comparisons between where I am and where I have been, but it is in these in-between moments when we are at our truest.

We walked through wide avenues made out of what appeared to be the riverbed's sand, and followed the music coming from the "Ras Lilas" (the love poems of Radha and Krishna) being performed in various ornately decorated camps along the road. The scene was strangely reminiscent of the American Old West, with its brightly lit facades set against relatively remote and vacant surroundings. Since our arrival at dusk, the temperature had dropped significantly. We were cold, and started to get headaches from the inhalation of dust and noise that encompassed us. We decided to head back to rest up for the morning's bath. That night I shivered myself into a deep sleep.

When we awoke at 6:00 A.M., the noise was nearly as loud as it had been the previous night. We wondered if it ever ceased. We dressed in our saris and headed out barefoot toward the sangam. It took us forty-five minutes, walking through endless crowds and over pontoons, to reach the main bathing area. The very public-private living of India was on display in every direction, with families gathered over food, men huddled around small fires, children sleeping, and babies being nursed. Everything here seemed communal.

We saw only a handful of other Westerners' faces along our final pilgrimage to the Kumbh. In the last stretch, we trudged in our saris through ankle-deep waters crowded with bathers, some praying quietly while others washed, bathed, or played, until we reached an area deep enough to submerge ourselves completely. This was the sacred place where this myth originated—Ganga and Yamuna, conjoined with the mythical Saraswati. Three divine life sources flowing gently together as millions of pilgrims did the same.

When it was my turn to dunk, I thought back to the adult baptism I had witnessed when I was confirmed as a Catholic. At that moment I marveled at this man's conscious choice to awaken his spirituality and commitment of faith. So I plunged into the murky waters three times, as I had the previous year in Haridwar, and I prayed for the people in Gujarat, my loved ones at home, and peace for the world. When I came up, I thanked God for this opportunity to experience life through this pilgrimage and for the reminder that I am awake, I am alive, and that I have the freedom to choose a spiritual path at the convergence of East and West.

Matsyasana

Matsya means "fish." This asana is dedicated to Matsya, the fish incarnation of the Hindu god Vishnu, a supreme deity and maintainer of the universe. In this pose, the chest and the head become the highest parts as the body, lying on the floor, forms an arch from the waist to the neck. The front of the body is fully extended and the chest completely expanded, facilitating breathing. The neck is well stretched, and results in the stimulation of the thyroid. Matsyasana also emphasizes the elasticity of the pelvic region.

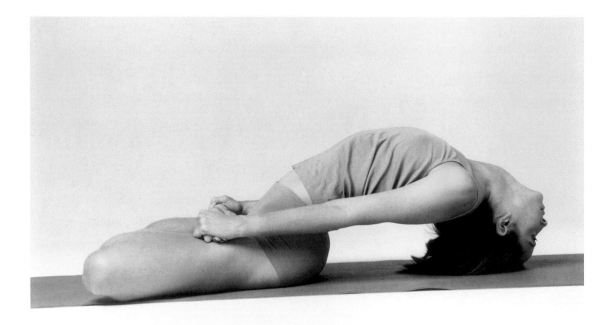

Balasana
(child's pose)

This pose, both physically and psychologically, represents a memory of ourselves as infants. Although it is physically less challenging than other poses, it forces the practitioner to confront a different challenge: to adopt a state of "non-doing" and to patiently surrender to gravity. The shape of Balasana requires the practitioner to breathe from somewhere other than the front of the lungs, which we are used to, by compressing the rib cage and abdomen against the thighs. Through this pose, we realize a different origin of our breath and begin to really tune in to a deeper, steadier breath. Balasana, practiced with a near-perfect breath (pranayama), pulls the energy of your breath behind the heart, the back of the lungs, across the chest, and around the organs. Resembling a child comfortable in the womb, this pose is an excellent stress-reliever and back pain alleviator. It is also recommended for relieving menstrual pain. A "wagging" version of the pose, which uses the motion of the chest against the thighs to massage the breast tissue and stimulate lymph flow, promotes breast health.

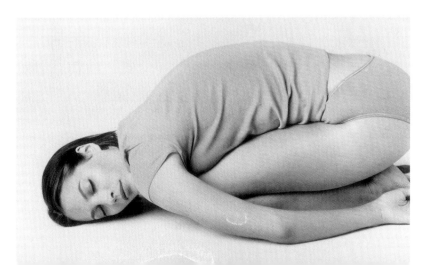

Padmasana
(lotus posture)

Padma means "lotus." *Asana* refers to pose. You may have heard its common name many times: Padmasana is commonly called the "lotus posture." It is also often

referred to as the "royal posture" or the "lotus throne," for with it the practitioner assumes a posture of beauty, grace, and divinity, much like the flower itself. The lotus is symbolic in many ways. It is a flower whose roots are in the mud, yet it grows up beyond the muddy water and floats on the surface of the water. It symbolizes the opposites of birth and death, male and female, and the interaction of the creative forces, according to *Hatha Yoga: The Hidden Language* by Swami Sivananda Radha.

The lotus has been considered the "Flower of Light," and has appeared in representations alongside gods of the Egyptians, Hindus, pagans, Chinese, and Buddhists, to name a few. Wherever it is found or placed, it immediately inspires an atmosphere of beauty and

sacredness. In Buddhism, the open lotus is associated with Buddha and heightened levels of consciousness, and the Buddha is often depicted sitting or standing on the flower. For both Buddhists and Hindus, the lotus symbolizes spiritual attainment and the flowering of human potential.

As the "lotus posture," padmasana often accompanies chanting and is the doorway to meditation. In this position, the legs are crossed, the feet resting on the thighs with the soles facing up, and the hands placed either on the knees, palms upward, or resting in the lap. It instinctively requires shifts in your body to achieve natural alignment and the erect spine maintains an alert and attentive, yet relaxed, mind. As with all asanas, the lotus posture has an effect on the glandular system. Medically speaking, the hands and feet contain more afferent and efferent nerves (sensory and motor, respectively), as well as endocrine glands, than any other single part of our body. When one sits in the lotus posture with legs crossed and hands folded, the bio-energy (which usually gets dissipated through our hands and feet) forms a closed circuit. The harnessing of this energy allows for greater attentiveness and deeper meditation. And though it is said to be the most ideal asana for higher meditation, do not be deceived by the easiness of its appearance—it may take some time and practice to learn to properly maintain the lotus posture in all of its forms.

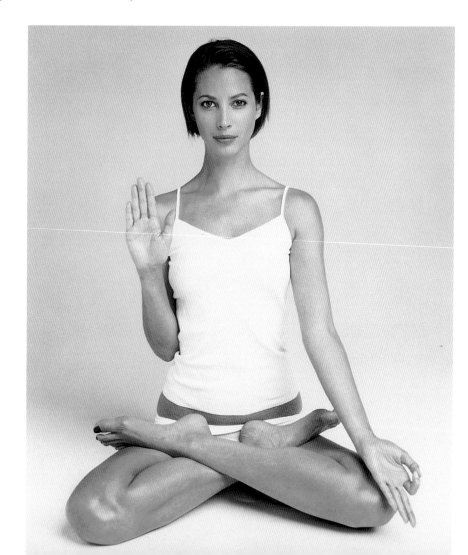

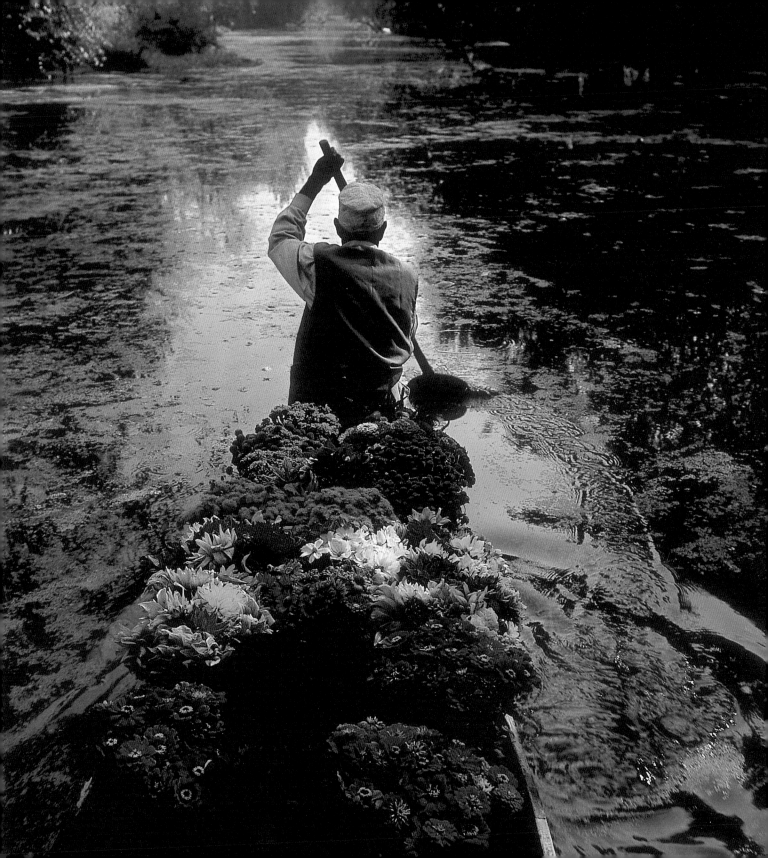

PERSONAL
JOURNEYS

INTENTIONS

"All limitations are self-imposed."

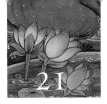

21

I believe that the experience of each moment presents

an opportunity for a new life. Many of us go through

the motions in life without fully realizing our poten-

tial for greatness, let alone true goodness or even

basic kindness. Passing routinely through the events

in one's lifetime, from one to the next without hon-

est reflection or examination of the meaning in them

and how each experience shapes us personally, denies

us that potential. We fill our days with commitments

and obligations to others, but often forget to think about ourselves. What about me? Focusing on the self may sound selfish or egocentric when, in truth, it can at times be one of the most generous things one can do for others. As we come to a deeper understanding of the self and our own actions, we are more likely to understand those of others. And in doing so, we are brought together in purpose and spirit, which ultimately defines the human condition.

An example of this within my own journey was when I decided to quit smoking. Only after making a serious commitment to myself was I able to make a serious commitment to quitting. I experienced firsthand the magnitude of my actions and how far-reaching they were, in that they not only affected me but those around me, as well. Almost immediately, my health and sense of well-being improved, which in turn allowed me to enjoy a greater quality of my life and my relationships. Also, quitting showed the people closest to me that I was committed to living a better and longer life, which would allow those relationships to further grow, flourish, and endure even the most challenging of circum-

stances. It also allowed me to show my peers and colleagues that I was extremely disciplined and determined; that I would not conform, nor would I stay within any kind of box. These small victories, which came as the result of one big victory, instilled in me a certain sense of invincibility. I chose to take this feeling as inspiration to become nobler in thought and deed. I then began to see my life as a sort of offering of good intentions . . . which led me back to yoga.

Often in a yoga class, there is a moment before the practice begins where everyone is invited to chant OM three times to cleanse the space and allow a pause between events, from where we have come and where we are going next. With this, we are reminded of our presence at that very moment. The yoga practice itself is in some way an excuse or at the least a platform to do so for a specified period of time. Each asana reminds us of the physical presence of our bodies and our shape at each moment, and as we shift from posture to posture, we maintain this awareness through alternating movement and stillness. There is a silent moment during practice where you can choose to dedicate your practice as an offering to someone or something that may need it. It is like a prayer or blessing for a loved one or cause other or higher than yourself, with you as the physical vehicle to deliver those efforts outside of yourself, beyond yourself. It is an act of generosity and love that, when combined, can be one of the most powerful energies in the universe. These moments of self-awareness and altruistic offerings are our intentions in yoga.

As a culture, we often make resolutions in the new year. We promise this and we give up that, but how much thought really goes into these pledges? How often are we simply acting out of habit or societal expectations? How long does it take before we fail to meet those promises? What are our chances for success? If a heightened awareness in what we say and do is the goal, then I suppose the promise itself is enough. After all, the intention is there. But what if we were all to make promises to ourselves and to others, and then actually fulfill them? Most of us want to be better people, don't we? Well, better is always within our reach.

An entry from my diary:

1-2-2002

Today is my thirty-third birthday. As I sit here in the cabin that my father built, with my family all around me, I am filled with gratitude. I am overwhelmed by beautiful memories of my father and childhood. I have heard many people speak of the pressures to have everything figured out by this age, if not just to merely be surviving. Perhaps those expectations are connected in some way to those examples of historical or spiritual characters such as Alexander the Great or Jesus Christ, even if only archetypically. Christ was just 33 when he was crucified on the cross 2002 years ago, dramatically affecting history and symbolically affecting every life since His own, even of those who don't believe in His being the true Christ and Savior. I think that we each desire to some degree to affect others beyond our own lifetimes, even if it does not extend beyond the lives of our own children. Positively influencing the lives of our own children would be enough—any life other than our own would be enough.

The first time I realized that, having affected my own life, I now wished to affect others' lives as well, I started the beginnings of another intention—to put to practical use what I knew and what I had experienced. After giving up smoking and losing my father to a smoking-related disease, which gave me the impetus to try to help others to quit smoking, I put myself out there with the intention to help at least one person through sharing my experience. For some of us, this is a natural instinct; for others, it must be awakened. The Dalai Lama says:

> Life becomes useful when you confront a difficulty; it provides a kind of value for your life to have the kind of responsibility to confront it and overcome it. Whereas if you do not feel such difficulties, there's no such responsibility, no role for you to play in your life . . . That challenge allows you to practice your ability. Basically, the purpose of life is to serve other people. From that point of view, a difficulty is really a great opportunity.

It is the challenges and the opportunities that they present that help us realize our intentions. They may vary from moment to moment, from day to day, but the more we seek a deeper understanding of ourselves, the greater the fulfillment we will find in our lives, in our relationships, and in our daily practice.

The Air We Share

Through an appreciation of our relationship with everything that is indeed a part of our reality, we increase our mindfulness of our expressions and ourselves. Consider the makeup of our bodies: We are made of the elements, microorganisms, flora, minerals, and so forth. A teacher once reminded me that the air we breathe is the same air that is breathed by all creatures, human and non-human, throughout all of time. He reminded me that I am breathing the same air that the dinosaurs once breathed. That very air is taken in by all living things, now and forever after. Because we are all so connected with the nature of reality and the reality of nature, it would be impossible to become truly mindful, truly at peace, and truly compassionate without linking our inner understanding of this with outer actions that reflect such insight. And how does that linking occur? Through yoking.

"When one tugs at a single thing in nature, he finds it attached to the rest of the world."
—JOHN MUIR

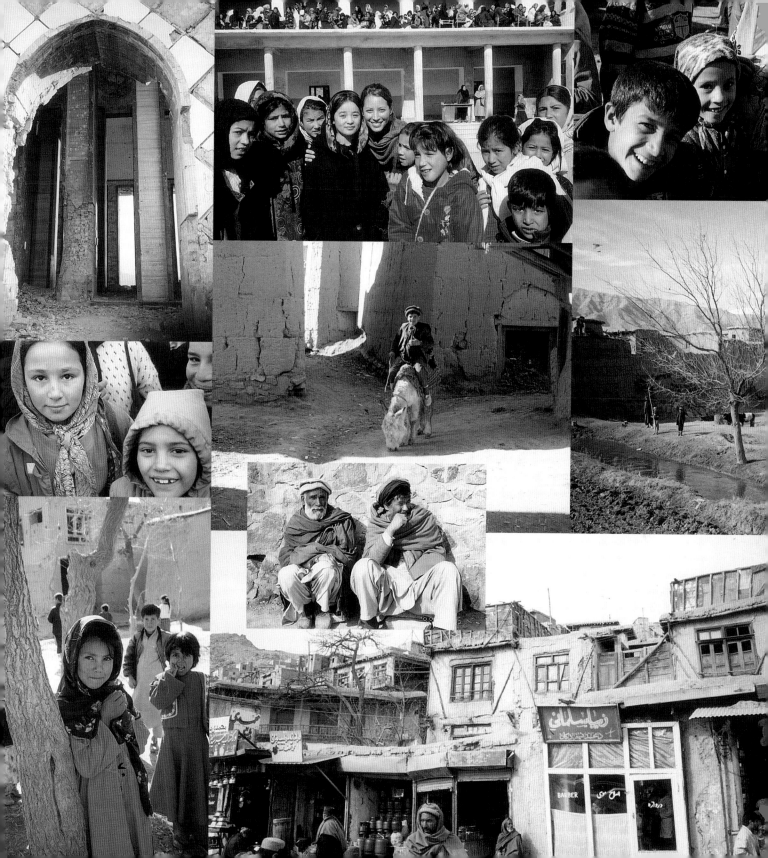

GLOBAL CONSCIOUSNESS

"The whole worth of a kind deed is in the love that inspires it."
—THE TALMUD

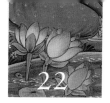

22

If you work hard toward becoming more open,

opportunities will beckon to you. If you are prepared,

profound experiences will occur deep within your

being. I have just returned from such a place, which

continues to provide just that type of experience.

Late last year, I received a call from a journalist

who asked if I would be interested in going to

Afghanistan. My curiosity immediately was piqued,

given the fragile state of affairs at that precise

moment. America had already been "at war" with Afghanistan for two months, in search of those allegedly responsible for what had occurred on September 11 in New York, which was targeted at the United States in particular and at the free Western world in general, for reasons not fully explained to or comprehended by the majority of its inhabitants on that day. "Yes," I said. "I am interested. When?"

It turned out that a national television network needed someone to do a follow-up story on the efforts of UNICEF on behalf of children throughout the region. We decided to angle our story on girls and young women, who were, for the first time in several years, now free to partake in their human right to receive an education along with males in the society.

We arrived in Kabul on January 20, 2002. I had gone there deliberately with little expectation, because I know how a place can change over time and with familiarity. Also, I don't watch a lot of mainstream television so as to preserve a somewhat unbiased opinion of world events, but these days it has been near-ly impossible to avoid all of the images and attitudes surrounding the events post–9/11. Coming from New York, the extremes between the ways of living were surreal. The population of Kabul hovers around four million. New York City's is seven and a half million. There are yellow taxicabs there, as well, but that is about the extent of comparability. Kabul is remarkably desolate, and feels more abandoned than inhabited. There are dwellings as far as the eye can see, but you have to wonder how they can be homes for people.

It was dark by 5:00 when we returned to our guesthouse for the night. As there isn't much to do in near-darkness, and I was tired, I turned in early for the night. The call to prayer from a nearby mosque became my internal clock. The same cue that awakens me is the one that summons me into bed until I can no longer keep my eyes open to read from *I Am That* by Sri Nisargadatta, a book lent to me by an Iranian friend of mine from home. I wrote down a quote from the book in my journal that first night that says: "Desire is the memory of pleasure and fear is the memory of pain."

The next morning, we went to visit nearby schools. We were pleasantly surprised to see hundreds of girls of all ages as they arrived. As they entered the school courtyard, smiling faces were revealed beneath the now infamously iconic blue burkas as they were immediately shed within the school's walls. I was instantly surrounded by small, beautiful, and inquisitive faces, each visibly overcome with joy and amazement. Many of them spoke at least some English, and took the opportunity to practice and engage with us. "Hello, what is your name?" they asked. "Salaam, my name is Christy," I responded. "What is your name?" I countered. "Welcome to our country," they said. "Where are you from?" they wanted to know. "America," I answered. "New York, USA." I looked for signs of contempt, but saw nothing but acknowledgment.

We visited classrooms filled with girls of various ages from grades one through six. Everyone would be given exams to determine what grade they were to be placed in when school began. I asked many of the girls what they wanted to be when they grew up. Almost everyone answered "doctor" or "teacher." When asked why, they said, "Because my country has many diseases and I would like to help my people," and, "Because I love my teacher and want to encourage others to learn."

At present, UNICEF is promoting a back-to-school campaign with an initiative geared toward equality called "Education for All." The goal is to send at least 1.5 million children back to school. Part of this initiative is to encourage female students to participate, rather than to attend passively. It is clear that discrimination against girls is the largest impediment to achieving this goal. Gender-sensitive classes should contain roughly equal numbers of girls and boys, and performance should ideally be at parity. Many girls drop out of school with the onset of menstruation, which makes them particularly vulnerable when there are no separate toilets to ensure privacy.

After our tour of several classrooms, we next visited a home school located across town and tucked away in a residential neighborhood. Some small schools like this remained open, despite numerous threats to close them if they did not comply and refuse girls. The teachers here told stories of warnings like this, and their refusal to adhere to such rules, no matter what the risk. I was filled with respect and awe at their courage and resilience. Later that evening, I was in bed and ready for sleep again by 7:00, my head and heart full of hope for this country and for the world. I wrote down this quote from my book before falling to sleep: "Want what you have, and care not for what you don't have."

We had met two sisters at the first school who spoke English well and had told us they had just returned home to Kabul from Peshawar, Pakistan, where they had been living for the last four years. They were enrolling in school when they saw us and approached us to ask for computers and better English teachers for their school. The eldest, Shahirzad, was fifteen. Shahirzad told me that she hoped to become a journalist because she wished to share with the world the plight of women's rights in Afghanistan. She was so eloquent about the situation in her country and passionate about her desire to change things to ensure a better future for her people. We spoke about September 11, which she was fully aware of, and she said that no life is worth causing an end to so abruptly or so maliciously. She said that she was deeply saddened to learn what had happened in my country, and that she was grateful for the concern from the outside world. She asked only that we do not forget the Afghan people again in the aftermath of this particular conflict. We were all so moved by this young woman, and when we left her at the school where we had accompanied her and her sister, sans burkas, we all knew we had caught a glimpse of the potential future of this country.

The final day was spent visiting sights around the city. Some were sites of heinous activity, alive only weeks ago, such as the stadium where women are routinely and publicly executed for senseless reasons. There were graveyards with freshly dug graves for the newly dead, some proudly staked with flags representing martyrs. We took a long drive out past the front lines and saw diligent roadside demining efforts on the way to a small village untouched by time.

While in Afghanistan, the majority of our contact was with children and old men. They were as intrigued with us as we were with them, and seemed honored when asked to have their picture taken. Everywhere we went, people returned our smiles, and oftentimes would place their right hand over their heart as a gesture of respect or acknowledgment. It was so new and beautiful to communicate so deeply without words. I saw my own eyes and smile on the faces of so many young girls throughout Kabul. They gave me hope when they had so little, which I tried to return to them. When you can see your own soul in another human being, you have attained yoga, and the world becomes an intimate place where your significance in it becomes clear again.

"All you need is to keep quietly alert, enquiring into the real nature of yourself.
This is the only way to peace."
—*I AM THAT* BY SRI NISARGADATTA MAHARAJ

ASH WEDNESDAY

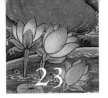

23

How appropriate for me that this year Ash Wednesday

fell on the day before Valentine's Day. Ash Wednesday

is a Christian holy day, followed by Lent, which com-

memorates the forty days that Jesus Christ spent wan-

dering in the desert. It leads up to Good Friday, when

He died on the cross. It is a time of penitence and

atonement. Faithful Christians go to mass on this day

to receive a blessing of ashes. These ashes are created

by burning the palm leaves from the previous year's

Palm Sunday Mass, which takes place a week before Easter, and are placed by a priest on the forehead in the sign of the cross.

I didn't start to participate in this holiday until adulthood, but I have grown to look forward to this six-week period of time as an excuse to withdraw a bit from the world and make a few sacrifices on behalf of my beliefs. Since visiting India and being inspired by the outward display of faith by Hindus with their *bindis* or *taliks,* Buddhists with their shaved heads and orange or purple robes, and Muslims with their covered heads, I really enjoy experiencing that single day in the year as a Catholic Christian when I can show off my faith, when others on the street or in the workplace look at you as an oddball. It sometimes amazes me how many Christians know so little about their own religion. I can only imagine that this is a common denominator among many of the others, as well.

Most years, on this particular day, I carry on with my life as usual, going to work and meetings with my ashes after mass. However, this year I was not feeling well, and called in sick. My extensive traveling of the past month had

suddenly caught up with me and I crashed. I spent the day resting, contemplating, and just being in my home again. I went to mass at 5:30 in the afternoon. Father Lafferty was presiding from the dais over a nearly full church. I love to attend afternoon masses in the wintertime. It is so warm and golden inside this sanctuary in contrast to the dark cold outside.

Father Lafferty walked up to the pulpit to deliver his homily in his usual warm way—with his kind face and gentle manner—and began to speak about the true meaning of Lent. He said that as we choose to sacrifice certain habits for Lent, we need to be sure that they are sacrifices for God, and not only for ourselves. Many Christians give up something for Lent. Typically it is alcohol, coffee, or sugar, or something similarly bad for us that we enjoy. It feels like a huge sacrifice, but it isn't really much of one at all because our intentions are misdirected. He told a story of a man who'd been on the Weight Watchers program all year long. The man confessed to him that it was so much easier to stay on the program during Lent. This implied that Lent was a time for him to recommit himself to his daily commitments, but not necessarily a time of sacrifice.

Most of us tend to choose things to give up that we know we can do without anyway. I know I do. I almost always give up alcohol, with the exception of when I gave up drinking for three years to help me quit smoking. This year, I had given up drinking alcohol and eating red meat . . . again. I had tried giving up the latter once before for a New Year's resolution a few years back, with the intention of slowly weaning myself off a meat-eating diet and easing into a vegetarian one. It was painless, so the following year I upped the ante and tried to cut out all poultry, too. The idea was to move down the food chain.

Let's not forget that none of these things I have mentioned are particularly healthy, and thus are also non-yogic, as we are told in many books and in the classroom. Ahimsa, the Hindu practice of non-violence, does not condone the eating of flesh in any form. Having grown up on a less restrictive American diet, I was accustomed to believing that I needed animal protein in my diet. I even craved meat upon occasion. But now that I was practicing

yoga more regularly, I wanted to overcome these conditioned cravings and to show more respect for other living creatures in their various forms. Besides, I argued to my carnivorous family and friends, how would I know if I really did need to eat meat (as the argument of most meat eaters goes) unless I gave it up? So I slid into vegetarianism as an experiment with my body. Now that I was more attuned to my physical body because of my yoga practice, I would let it tell me what it wanted or when certain nutrients were needed.

Things as a non-meat eater went smoothly for several months, as I ate only fish and vegetables. One day in the summer, however, I was out at some friends' beach house for a barbecue. They had been kind enough to consider my new stance and had bought some fish for me, and steak for the rest of the guests. I had hardly even thought about steak for the last year and a half, but now the smell of the marinated meat was too delicious to refuse. Like some sort of addict, I had one taste and I was off the vegetarian wagon. I felt so full of shame and failure, just as I had when trying to give up cigarettes years before and had relapsed. It was as if I'd taken two steps forward to fall one giant step behind again. Then I remembered that this had only been an experiment. I had to remind myself what I had told myself and others—that I would let my body tell me what it wanted or needed. For whatever reasons, at that point it wanted meat.

The way I was feeling about myself after falling from grace was certainly not yogic, that's for sure. I confided to a yogi friend about what I was going through, and he warned me to try to avoid being rigid. He reminded me that we all need to be more gentle and forgiving with ourselves. When we examine our frustration at not being able to maintain discipline and our sense of defeat, we need to step back and either start over, or resolve the inner conflict that we are experiencing.

This perspective has been an important lesson for me in my practice, and one that continues to challenge me. It may take some time to live the way we think we want to live. And on the way, we may also discover that the path we are on is not necessarily the exact way for us. As we feed ourselves physically, we can remember to be mindful of the food that we eat and all that we choose to put into our bodies for nourishment. And when feeding ourselves mentally, pausing before a meal to give thanks is enough for a start. To be thankful for all that went into a meal, the sacrifice of an animal's life perhaps, the work in preparation and presentation, the care and the love if it is home cooked, is enough. But if not red meat, what then do we give up for Lent that is meaningful?

What is bad about particular vices such as coffee, alcohol, and tobacco is not so much that they are very bad for your health—which they certainly are, as Father Lafferty confirmed from the pulpit—but that they obscure your reality and the truth. During the Lenten time, which is meant to bring us closer to God, clarity is what we need most of all. We need to create a quiet place within ourselves to have that dialogue with God. Many religions abstain from many or all of these substances at all times, particularly the religions that require the outwardly visible signs of faith that I mentioned earlier. These faiths encourage meditation, prayer, and contemplation on a daily basis.

For me as a Catholic, one day in particular reminds me of these needs. Ash Wednesday is a time to contemplate the life of Jesus Christ and His sacrifice for us Christians, but it is also a time to recognize the value of life, as you might if you had to spend forty days alone in the desert. You would probably come out of the desert knowing yourself quite well. You would also probably emerge with a lot of ideas about how you want to live your life, or how you can better the one that you have. You don't have to be Christian to practice sacrific-ing the things that keep you from your Self. Try giving up those things in your life that distract you from you, and open your heart to the things that will reveal you to you.

So for me, this year I promised myself that Lent would be a time of contemplation, free of travel for work, and avoiding days packed without spaces to pause in between. It is a time to go inward, to work on my home, and to focus on my relationships and on myself.

A DAY DEDICATED
TO THE HEART

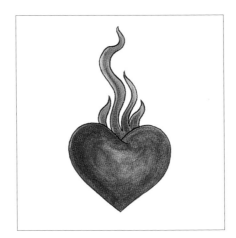

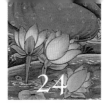

24

Valentine's Day. What is it really about? The origin is not entirely clear, but it is considered to be in commemoration of St. Valentine, a Christian martyr who died in the year 269. Prior to his martyrdom, he was a priest in Rome who assisted martyrs during the persecution under Emperor Claudius II. He was arrested for his actions and when he refused to renounce his faith, he was beaten and beheaded. He proved that he was a true servant of God by offering his compassion to others and by his willingness to die for his beliefs. So, each year, when so many of us buy cards and gifts decorated with hearts and cupids for our loved ones, it is compassion that is to be celebrated. Compassion is a vehicle for love and a channel for gratitude. Often this day is a day of showing our appreciation for others, which is in and of itself a form of gratitude. But it can also be a day to appreciate ourselves too.

I started Valentine's Day this year recording a poem written by Deepak Chopra and inspired by the love poems of Rabindranath Tagore for a CD. I was asked by Deepak to contribute to this project by reading a poem, and unconsciously somehow, the day I chose to read fell on this day, the day of the heart. Each person participating was invited to read a poem from his selected collection. I chose a poem entitled "Be." I had very little time to prepare prior to the recording but, while reading it aloud, I realized why I had chosen it. There are no accidents.

Spells, charms, incantations
There is nothing left to say
The magic of music enfolds intention
Centuries of knowledge

Layers of experience, an entire history
In a few melodies

Our lifetime is packaged inside of us
As imprints triggered by lyric
Wrapped in words the way a
Spider wraps flies in a gossamer
We are both the spider and the fly
Imprisoned and free in our own web

When I say that there are no accidents, I mean to say that when you are open, you find the message in just about everything that echoes perfectly for where you are on your spiritual path. For me, there are many lessons to be found in this poem. The first word that struck me was *intention*. It is a word that I use a lot, and am constantly mindful of. I use it because it reflects my desire, or intention rather, to be mindful of everything that I do. Intention is what is required in order to do that. However, I have often made lifestyle choices for myself that leave little time for such thought and care.

This poem speaks to me of the knowledge that the whole of the world is inside each and every one of us, waiting to be awakened. It also likens life to music, which is often at its most beautiful when it is complex, like a symphony or great jazz. Language does not always capture the subtleties of experience. We inherently have the capacity for truth, yet we often tend to trap ourselves with false promises contradictory to that truth. The last line of the poem is especially powerful, as it reminds me of the saying that freedom is a state of mind. This is something that is very hard to fully comprehend, and even harder to put into practice.

Nelson Mandela is one such man who came to understand this through experience. He spent nearly a lifetime in prison on a small island in South Africa in virtual exile from his country and people, for which he fought, and which led him to the place where he was. He came to know his inner world as a paradise, unmoved by the reality that was his external world. Through his experience alone, we can almost understand the lesson of his life. If we meditate on his experience, for example, it may be easier to consider living our lives differently, or, at least, more mindfully.

When I was finished recording my poem on Valentine's Day, I felt charged with positive reinforcement from my small audience of producer and sound engineer, and from myself, as well. It felt good to partake in this project, to give voice and speak emotion to the written word so that others might in turn find their own meanings in these profound truths. I was compelled to hug each person in the room, though I had only just met them. I wished them all a happy Valentine's Day and was off again.

Normally, my days do not start so smoothly. I am usually rushing from one appointment to the other. I find that it is important to set a tone at the beginning of a day, as early as possible, so that it can hopefully carry consistently throughout. Though it may not always happen, this is a personal goal of mine, nonetheless. I thought that that day was a good day to set a special tone—to practice compassion for myself.

I arrived at my next appointment, at NBC, early! I emphasize this because it *never* happens. And so I relished the opportunity to pause in the lobby of the enormous office building and actually *wait* for my producer to escort me upstairs to track my voice for the story on Afghanistan. I had been there a few days before to see the rough cut of the piece and to receive a little tutelage from a broadcaster, since this was not my profession. I had taken the time to prepare myself; more so than usual because I wanted to do my very best. It can be a little daunting to put yourself into a position that is unfamiliar. Accepting this project was a challenge, and since then I've been practicing taking my commitments more seriously.

There, while reading through the script, having practiced and feeling more comfortable with the dialogue that would be laid over the film footage I had experienced and had now seen in its nearly completed form, I was again uplifted internally, just as I had been an hour before. My performance was appreciated, and I felt reassured that this important story would bring about an awareness for millions of people who might not have had it otherwise. The people in our story were to have a reach beyond their wildest expectations through this medium. As we watched the segment again, I was happy to see how eloquent they were, because this would help demystify their culture to ours. So far, this day was turning out to be one of the best I could recall, and I was mindful and grateful that I could acknowledge that while still experiencing it.

Outside, it was a cold but sunny day. As I rode downtown in the back of a cab, I looked out the window rather than down at my work, or phone, or computer. I took the twenty-minute ride as another opportunity to pause between events. Though I arrived a bit late for my next appointment, I was calmer than usual. The rest of my will was to be spent on my new home.

When I arrived at the space, still in a state of construction, there were workmen everywhere. This is what a homeowner likes to see on an unannounced visit! I was there for a Vastu consultation with expert Kathleen Cox. My intention was to create a home that would be a source of personal empowerment, as well as a haven from the world—a sacred space. Though Vastu comes from Vedic science, which can seem very complex at first, it involves a lot of common sense and is easy to integrate into your life in a way that suits and nourishes your lifestyle. We found a room in the southeast corner of the apartment with a dusty table and less noise for our session. While waiting for me, Kathleen took some time familiarizing herself with the space. She then explained many of the practical aspects and applications of Vastu. At the end of our brief session, Kathleen reiterated my lesson for the day: "Just be mindful of every choice, for that is what Vastu achieves." With this lingering in my head, I gave Kathleen a big hug and expressed my gratitude for her help before heading back to my current home to work with my architect and designer, dear friends of mine who had been living with me since September 11, to integrate my Vastu lessons into the plan. Sitting in my living room that evening, I realized that, as the saying goes, home is truly where the heart is. But I still like the idea of creating a new home that expresses my heart, too. The lesson of the day is, "Start with the heart." This is the way to strive to begin each and every day.

Rabindranath Tagore

Rabindranath Tagore was born to a Hindu family in Bengal in 1861. Educated in Bengal and in England, he experienced early success as a writer and soon gained wide popularity in the West, as well. He became known as the voice of India's spiritual heritage and, though he was a writer of all genres, including music, his poetry made him a living institution. A friend of Gandhi and a major voice in the social, political, and cultural movements in early twentieth-century India, Tagore won the Nobel Prize for literature in 1913 for his poetry. He died in 1941.

NON-ATTACHMENT

"Nothing can bring you peace but yourself.
Nothing can bring you peace but the triumph of principles."
—RALPH WALDO EMERSON

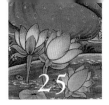

25

I was starting to feel that I had really begun to

understand the Buddhist theory of non-attachment,

until September 11. Sure, I like the artifacts and

mementos I have accumulated through my travels,

and there are certainly some things I prefer to others,

but I believe I can truthfully say that I do not own a

single thing I could not live without. Anything I have

ever lost, I have learned to live without. Of course, it

feels liberating to realize this but, naturally, you can

never know exactly how you will feel until you find yourself there, alone with just yourself.

My wedding date was only weeks away from that glorious but fateful autumn morning in Manhattan. My entire family was in New York visiting because there were all sorts of festivities planned for the bride. Friends from every life I have lived so far were there to celebrate me and my future life. I had been planning the wedding for nearly nine months, the length of a pregnancy term, and was taking it almost as seriously. The wedding took on a life of its own, but first had to take a number, just the same, along with the rest of my projects. I had never imagined one specific kind of wedding, but somehow the event was shaping itself into a dream wedding, despite the typical nightmares that were sure to accompany it.

As with any wedding, there was so much to do. However, as I have a habit of doing, I had to make it even more challenging for myself. To start with, I chose to marry outside of the country. This was supposed to keep the ceremony intimate, but there were all sorts of unforeseen formalities in doing so. I wanted a

Catholic wedding, and we wanted our priest in New York to come over with us to make it all the more meaningful. We decided to design our own rings so that they would be truly one of a kind, which meant additional meetings. Luckily, some friends offered their home for the reception, which alleviated some of the stress. Eventually, and possibly miraculously, all of the elements were in place. It was going be perfect, and that is what I had become attached to.

Along the way, I had some help; but, as the saying goes, if you want something done right, you should do it yourself. I felt that nobody, in terms of my wedding, could do things as well as I could. Over the summer, my fiancé and I had gone through Pre-Cana with the priest at our parish to prepare for the holy sacrament of marriage in the Catholic tradition. This would be the first marriage for us both, and we wanted to be prepared. All that remained was choosing the readings from the Bible and a poem for our program to send off for printing. We chose a poem written by the Sufi mystic Rumi. Of course, there were some tense times—would I keep my father's name, would I sign a pre-nuptial agreement that put pressure on our future happiness? All the while, we were looking for a place to live together. It was a lot to deal with, but I willed it away for the time being. I hid it all under the veil of my ego, and besides, there was hardly time for doubt now anyway. And then September 11 happened, seemingly out of nowhere at first.

That month, Pattabhi Jois was visiting from Mysore, India, to lead an Astanga workshop, which had been moved from one location to another for the week. I was coming down with a little something following the long celebratory weekend, so I had skipped the workshop on Monday.

It was still dark when I awoke at 5:30 A.M. Tuesday morning. I walked the dog and then sat waiting on my stoop for friends to collect me. We drove across quiet, empty West Village streets and up through Chelsea till we arrived at the piers. Dozens of yogis gathered in the Chelsea Piers gymnasium, a cold contrast to the warm, spacious loft in the Puck building, where classes had been held the previous week.

Fluorescent lights loomed far overhead while we yogis took our seats and chatted quietly or stretched atop the slick, shiny basketball court floor. A quiet hush arrived like a wave on a shore as a presence as graceful as water glided over each neat row of bodies. Everyone waited obediently for their guru's cue. Class began with the usual invocation to Patanjali, the guru's guru's guru, and then we were led, Mysore-style, through the series following his own long irregular counting. An hour and a half later, at 8:00 A.M., we slowly arose from our lying savasana poses and lined up to pay homage to the guru before beginning our days. When we drove out of the parking lot and into the sunshine outside, we turned out onto the West Side Highway and headed south directly toward the World Trade Center.

I arrived home at 8:30 A.M., and had an hour to kill before my first appointment of the day. I changed my clothes and sat with my mother over a cup of tea. We were watching the *Today Show* together when the program was interrupted by a news flash: A low-flying plane had just crashed into one of the Twin Towers.

People who had witnessed the crash were calling in from various locations in lower Manhattan to tell the reporter what they could see. Nobody seemed to think that the plane was a commercial jet, but everyone wondered how, on such a magnificent day, a pilot could not have seen where he was headed. Smoke billowed from the windows of the building.

We sat stunned as we watched and listened to the panicked reports, mere blocks away from where we were. My fiancé lives only eight short blocks from what would from then on be referred to as Ground Zero, and he was somewhere down in that area when the second plane hit the first tower's twin. Speculation that this was an act of terrorism escalated by the minute, but still I was not convinced. The phone rang, and it was my fiancé. He was safe in his living room, gazing horrified at what appeared to be bodies falling through the windows of the Towers. We hung up and I left for my next appointment, thinking that whatever the reason behind this was, it would take at least the rest of the day for it to begin to be clarified.

I walked up Sixth Avenue looking over my shoulder the whole of the eleven blocks from my house, back toward the Towers as they both streamed smoke. Now the sirens of fire trucks and police cars could be heard coming from every direction and heading toward them. I stepped into my appointment at 9:30 and reemerged forty-five minutes later to learn that the Pentagon had also been hit, and that several more planes were reported to be in the air with terrorists on board. I left and walked back to Sixth Avenue. When I turned the corner, I saw that the World Trade Center had disappeared.

As I walked, in shock, I passed dozens of people heading north, away from the disaster. Traffic had come to an absolute halt, and many people were huddled in small clusters, listening to car radios through doors left ajar. Others were crying or describing to one another what they had witnessed with their own eyes. All pay phones were in use, and everyone who had a cell phone was on it (though nearly all service had been disrupted). I could not believe that the Towers had fallen so quickly. Years and years of erecting these giants, down in only seconds. Had I not been certain that I had seen them earlier that morning, I'd have thought they were never even there in the first place.

When I reached my corner, I turned right and saw that a line of blood donors had already assembled down the block from the hospital on the opposite corner. Everyone in my house was awake, anxious, and glued to the news when I reached the house. My business partners and I sent all employees home from our SoHo offices before the area was officially evacuated. My nieces continued to play, joyfully ignorant beside distraught friends who had come over with their infant son, my godchild, to escape the hysteria in TriBeCa. They could not find their brother, who lived even nearer to the site, along with his wife and two sons. Only now did I wonder where my fiancé was, and began to fear the possibility of something having happened to him since we'd spoken. The phone was useless, as all circuits were busy. All we could do was sit and wait as the television frenzy intensified. It was hours before he turned up, along with my brother-in-law, who had gone down to search for him.

They had crossed over to the West Side Highway and had purchased water on the way.

By the afternoon, the hospital next door was packed with media and families searching for loved ones and friends. People began posting homemade signs all over the neighborhood, with photocopied pictures and personal information about the missing; those who had worked in or near the Towers and had not yet been seen or heard from. The streets had been closed below Fourteenth Street, so there was an eerie, peaceful, silent backdrop to the still-screaming sirens that had begun hours before. Neighbors were gathered in clusters outside, comparing stories and plotting escapes out of the city. Bridges, tunnels, subways, and buses were all closed, and people felt trapped. You could read on their faces that their imaginations were taking over. The air around the city was thick with fear and death.

I withdrew from the external chaos around me and fell into a deep, coma-like slumber while the television blared on. My immediate concern was that this horrific incident would fuel an open season for hate crimes and more unnecessary racial bias around the country and the world. I feared what might happen to non-extremist Muslims, who make up the majority of that religious population. Fear is debilitating on every level. The news was already recirculating itself by evening, bombarding us with terrifying imagery and encouraging public paranoia, and continued for several days doing the same.

I went to mass on Wednesday, partly to pray and partly for something to do; to get out of the house and see people other than my own family. It was difficult not to feel guilty and helpless in the wake of such grief. At the same time, we were experiencing a taste of collective consciousness seemingly so rare in our culture, which too often cultivates separatism and isolation amongst us. Walking back from church, I noticed the visages of each person that I passed. Things were different. There was solidarity in the air. People were more patient than usual when interacting, more sincere. Everyone in the neighborhood was walking in the middle of the streets, which were still free of cars, at drastically slowed down paces. It was as if some spell had been cast

over the entire island of Manhattan to make everyone's behavior markedly changed. It was a sad yet magical time to be alive.

The air outside was worsening, but we could no longer just sit indoors watching the kids climb the walls. We sent my family ahead to the beach in Long Island to stay with friends, where we met them the following afternoon. The bridges had reopened, and the scene that followed looked like a mass exodus out of the city—destination: anywhere. The journey that normally took two and a half hours took close to five.

It was hard to leave the city. As soon as we got out, I suddenly wanted back in. I felt disconnected from myself somehow, like a separation anxiety. The city seemed to pull on my heart, turning my attention far away from my relatively small "inner sanctum." Something was gently and relentlessly tugging at my compassion.

Over the weekend, I considered the personal ramifications of this atrocity. My business partners and I were just about ready to leave for Europe to launch our product line in several cities, then I was due in Germany for a meeting for another project before going to the destination of my wedding. I had been planning to not return home for a long time, because we'd intended to enjoy an extended honeymoon that involved a great amount of international travel.

Everything had been so tightly planned that there was wasn't any room for surprises. I am a planner to a fault. A true Capricornian "control freak," I always say, unapologetically, that I am simply not spontaneous. The truth is, planners leave little space for spontaneity because we fear it. On September 11, though, I found myself and my plans out of my control. The airports were closed, so travel did not seem possible for the immediate future. This created a domino effect and I lost further control, as there was no room to push back even one previously scheduled moment in my grand plan. Then, when somebody asked the inevitable question, "Will you go on with the wedding?" I responded without giving it a moment's thought, "Yes." Later, however, my fiancé

and I agreed that it was too early to make that call.

In the meantime, we did alter our honeymoon plans to avoid the potentially dangerous locations in light of the alleged groups suspected to be responsible for the attacks. My feelings were more than mixed about all of this. I did not want to stop my life and go on living in fear of potential dangers that may still be impossible to avoid, yet I had to think of others and their safety, too. I alerted everyone to the possibility of reconsidering our plans, given the state of the world. People were genuinely sympathetic and patient, allowing me some time to decide. After a few days back at work and a few conversations later with friends and family, we decided to proceed as planned. Until America began bombing Afghanistan, I was away on location, on a photo shoot. I had expected the day would come, so was not surprised, as so many seemed to be. It was just one week from our intended departure date for our wedding.

When I finally had a chance to speak with my fiancé from the airport on my way home, he asked me if I was aware of what was going on in the world.

"Yes," I said, "of course."

He said, "Well, then. What should we do?"

"What do you mean, what should we do?" I challenged him.

He then went on to tell me that he had spoken to almost everyone on his side of our guest list, who had all called him asking whether or not we were going to cancel. "Haven't you heard from any of your friends?"

"No," I said defiantly. "We need to talk about this."

"My friends have all canceled, and my family isn't too thrilled about flying abroad, either," he said.

Now, so close to leaving, my fiancé was basically telling me that we were not going to go through with the plans we'd made. He wanted to talk about it, but there was no point. I needed to give people the notice they would need to stop the wheels already in motion. I immediately sent e-mails to everyone invited, letting them know what was decided. I was angry at those who had started this mess, and angry at our government for retaliating, and I was angry at my fiancé for giving up so easily. The truth is, it was nobody's fault, and I needed to get over myself.

When it was suggested that we relocate the ceremony, I refused. No matter where we chose, some people would still have to travel, so if this was our reason for postponing, then we would have to wait until it was safe for everyone. Of course, there is the possibility that such a time may never come. Some people in this country will never travel again. Others may never travel abroad, and some, like myself, who travel for a living, will have to overcome whatever natural fears they have. Fortunately, time is a magnificent healer because it allows a perspective from a situation that only distance can provide; a chance to realize that there are reasons for every action.

This is where non-attachment comes in. Seeing yourself as a part of an experience but not the experience itself, allows you to stay flexible and liberates you from outcomes you cannot control. When things larger than yourself happen in the universe, it is important to honor them and all of their reverberations. Take this opportunity to take account of all the many things you have to be grateful for, and know that the universe will take care of you when you are ready to begin again.

BE HERE NOW,
WHEREVER YOU ARE

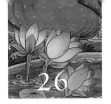

A few years ago, I read a book called *The Bonds of Love* by Jessica Benjamin. I was especially intrigued by one particular chapter that went into a discourse on the inequality of the sexes. Benjamin theorized that because men were traditionally considered the "doers" and women the "be-ers," for children today, these notions were perpetuating a detriment in our culture. Basically, in families with two parents, children learn through the observation of both individuals and their respective behavior. If only one parent works, the children may regard that parent as the autonomous one and the other as the more passive antithesis. Likewise, if there is only one parent, this individual has the potentially greater challenge to meet all the needs of her child or children at once. Needless to say, we must constantly reevaluate and question the "role" of roles because there are so many factors involved in creating a family.

In my family, it was my father who worked while my mother stayed home with my sisters and me. As a small child, I regarded my father as the doer because he was off "doing" —working to provide for all of us. While my father was away working, my mother cared for us, looking after our needs, "being" there for us to nurture and instill a sense of stability. Looking back, I can now see their partnership as the combination relationship required to create this balance; but for a long time, all I wanted was to be more like him and less like her. I don't think that this choice had as much to do with my parents and who they were as people per se, but was more likely tied to their designated roles within our family and maybe even to their comfort levels within those roles

that influenced my decisions early on in how I would live my life.

The result of that early choice is a life that has thus far been largely spent "doing," and far too little of it just "being." When I was younger, the two roles seemed to contradict each other because they were dichotomized into responsibilities, as opposed to showing two people with different natures integrated into one role with many responsibilities and reinforcement for us, their pupils. In retrospect, I would say that my twenties were spent establishing a path for myself that was to be acknowledged by others, albeit slightly out of order, since work came before school (we usually believe, sometimes falsely, that the degree must precede the recognition). Years later, I am spending my early thirties in catch-up mode, because of my late start. I am now guilty of having gained enough acknowledgment from the world, yet still I find myself working for it. This is my thirty-third year and I am on the cusp of another major transition. On my birthday this year, I decided that I would dedicate the rest of my thirties, and my life, for that matter, to work on myself. If I practice "being" now, I will cultivate that much more to my Self and those with whom I come into contact in the future.

When I started a regular asana practice, it became abundantly clear that I was only using one tenth of my energy capacity in this world. By capacity, I am referring to strength, endurance, concentration, flexibility, and breath, not to mention brainpower. Through my practice, I began to utilize far more of myself and came to rely on myself more than on others. For a "doer," however, expanding your capacity can be dangerous, too, because it allows the "doer" to "do" more, as in my case.

Suddenly, I found myself taking on more and more. So much so, that even my yoga practice seemed like work and left me feeling drained. Eventually, all of this productivity proved to be counterproductive. The more energy you cultivate, the more you feel you have to expend. Not true. Most of the energy you cultivate is, in fact, energy you need to sustain yourself. I had been running on depleted energy for so long that I ended up feeling completely out of balance with the new surplus I had attained. I soon learned that energy, like money, is easier to make than to save.

In the last couple of years, I have learned an important lesson: Just because I *can* (do something), doesn't mean that I *should*. This is quickly becoming a mantra of mine because of its relevance to practically everything that I take on. But, sometimes just knowing something isn't enough to make it a reality for us, is it? I am in a fortunate position in life. This, I am sure of. We make choices throughout our lives that will continue to affect us as long as we live. Each choice opens the door to more choices, and so on. But, because I am a seeker and am open and drawn to new experiences, experiences seek me out as well. To make the best choices for ourselves, we need to know ourselves deeply so that we can live joyfully with our decisions long after the moment of truth. After all, "the truth will set us free."

A key element to creating a life practice is realizing that "being" isn't as passive as we may think. Anyone who has tried to sit and practice meditation will tell you that the mind is far more active than we as physical entities could ever be. The mind tricks us into believing that we can keep up with it when it is, in actuality, impossible. I am constantly surprised each and every time someone asks me if asana practice is really all that challenging for my body. People confuse meditation with physical yoga all the time, and while they are mutually beneficial, they are also independent and individually complex paths. Some postures are not only incredibly physically challenging, but are mentally challenging, as well. It really makes no difference whether you are naturally flexible or not, because the practice asks you to find that movement through the breath at your furthest point.

Most of all, yoga brings you back to the present, time and time again. If you are breathing correctly and following the breath in your postures with each inhalation and exhalation, you will find yourself present. Being is presence. There is a well-known book, *Be Here Now* by Ram Dass, whose title is a reminder that all we truly have are the moments that we are in. Not much else is as relevant. Sure, our families and people matter, but without our true presence, we are of little use to anyone else. And, if each moment is carefully considered, the past and future will bring less worry back our way today.

We all know that worrying doesn't solve anything. In fact, it is almost like praying for bad things to happen. For those things that keep coming back to you through memory or worry: The time is now. There is an expression that says: "Wherever you go, there you are." What this says to me is that there is no external escaping the stuff in our minds. Peace of mind can only come from practicing the quieting of the mind and observing yourself in each moment.

"Doing" is oftentimes running from your self and preoccupying your mind and body with distractions from the self. Our goal should be to attain a sort of effortless effort through our actions that will bring us back to our most honorable selves. We need work only to provide for our families and ourselves. And going about our work with a certain level of mindfulness is essential. When we lose sight of what we are working for, it becomes "destructive doing." We can also choose to serve God through our work, no matter what our job, as the dedication of our efforts can be what is offered up. If we can get ourselves to a state of "being while doing," or even to recognize that being *is* doing, we will have successfully integrated these two natures and will be able to experience the harmony.

Yoga, Bhakti Yoga, and Jnana Yoga

japa—repetition of mantra

jiva—life, the individual soul, or essence

jivamukti—the liberation of one's essence

Jnana Yoga—a system of yoga that emphasizes inquiry and insight

Karma Yoga—the path of yoga based on action that encourages detachment from results and emphasizes selfless behavior

kriya—action, or practice

kundalini—the obstacle located at the base chakra that blocks the upward flow of prana, the kundalini is often depicted as a coiled serpent

Mahabharata—the epic poem written sometime between 500 B.C.E. and 300 B.C.E. in which the Bhagavad Gita is inserted

Mahayana—the school of Buddhism that promotes the "bodhisattva" ideal—the renunciation of personal liberation to stay in this world and be dedicated to helping others

mandala—a spiritual diagram offering a symbolic representation of the universe, incorporating sacred geometry, often used as a visual aid for meditation

mantra—a sacred sound or word often used as a tool in meditation

moksha—liberation, same as mukti

mudra—symbol; in Yoga, a symbolic gesture

nadi—a channel through which prana flows within the subtle body

niyama—personal attitude, discipline; the second limb of astanga

OM—the primordial sound, one of the most sacred mantras

padma—lotus

padmasana—the lotus posture

Panini—a Hindu scholar credited with codifying Sanskrit

Patanjali—the author of the *Yoga Sutras*

prakrti—nature, cosmic manifestation

prana—life force, breath

pranayama—breath control, the fourth limb of astanga

pratyahara—sense withdrawal, the fifth limb of astanga

purusha—spirit, or unseen energy

Raja Yoga—a system of yoga that incorporates the eight limbs but whose emphasis is on meditation

sadhana—personal practice

samadhi—deep concentration, liberation, the eighth limb of astanga

Sanskrit—the sacred language of India and of Yoga

satsang—a religious gathering centered around a spiritual guide

shakti—spiritual energy or power

siddha—a liberated being, a perfected yogi

Surynamaskara—a specific sequence of asanas known as the "sun salutation"

sutra—thread

tantra—technique

Tantra Yoga—a system of yoga that emphasizes the unblocking of prana through practices that are often disregarded by other yogic systems

tapas—purification, austerity

ujjayi—the victorious breath, a pranayama technique that focuses on the evenness and sounds of forceful breathing (often used in Astanga Yoga)

Upanishads—the mystical teachings of the end of the Vedas, from which the foundation for Hinduism was laid

Vedanta—"the end of the Veda," a designation for the Upanishads

Vedas—"knowledge," the collection of spiritual hymns of divine revelation that provide the earliest known mentionings on Yoga, thus forming the very first basis for the philosophy

vinyasa—the fluid sequence of postures, "breath-synchronized movement"

Vishnu—one of the gods of the Hindu Trinity, known for his creative potency and many reincarnations

yama—our attitudes to our environment and the world, the first limb of astanga, self-control

yoga sadhana—yoga practice

yogi—one who practices yoga

Some information in this glossary is from *A Popular Dictionary of Hinduism* by Karel Werner (Chicago: NTC Publishing Group, 1997).

ENDNOTES

(p. 27.) Georg Feuerstein, Ph.D., *The Yoga Tradition: Its History, Literature, Philosophy and Practice* (Prescott, AZ: Hohm Press, 1998), p. 5.

(p. 34.) T. K. V. Desikachar, *Health, Healing & Beyond: Yoga and the Living Tradition of Krishnamacharya* (New York: Aperture, 1998), p. 55.

(p. 46.) Sri K. Pattabhi Jois, *Yoga Mala* (New York: Eddie Stern, 1999), p. 15.

(p. 53.) Bikram Choudry, *Beginning Yoga Class* (New York: Tarcher Putnam, 1978), p. 57.

(p. 70.) Rinpoche quote from Rudolph Wurlitzer, *Hard Travel to Sacred Places* (Boston: Shambhala, 1995), pp. 108–109.

(p. 70.) John McAfee, *The Fabric of Self* (Colorado: Woodland Publications, 2001), p. 55.

(p. 78.) B. K. S. Iyengar, *Light on Pranayama* (The Crossroad Publishing Company, 2001), xvii and (second quote on that page) xxi.

(p. 84.) *The Hatha Yoga Pradipika* (ancient text), Chapter 2, S.3.

(p. 94.) Jane Hope, *The Secret Language of the Soul: A Visual Guide to the Spiritual World* (San Francisco: Chronicle Books, 1997), p. 140.

(p. 8.) David Fontana, *The Secret Language of Symbols: A Visual Key to Symbols and Their Meanings* (San Francisco: Chronicle Books, 1994), p. xxxx, 13.

(p. 100.) Yogi Bhajan, *The Teachings of Yogi Bhajan* (Arcline Publications, 1977), pp. 3–4.

(p. 146.) McAfee, p. 96.

(p. 182.) Kathleen Cox, *Vastu Living: Creating a Home for the Soul* (New York: Marlowe & Co., 2000); also in personal interview.

(p. 198-99.) Ernest Hemingway, *The Snows of Kilimanjaro* (New York: Charles Scribner & Sons, 1995), p. 27.

(p. 101.) Feuerstein, p. 236.

(p. 166.) Geeta S. Iyengar, *Yoga: A Gem for Women* (Spokane, WA: Timeless Books, 1990), p. 169.

(p. 216.) Swami Sivananda Radha, *Hatha Yoga: The Hidden Language* (Spokane, WA: Timeless Books, 1995), p. 121.

(p. 116.) *Yoga Journal*, October 2001, article archive from Yoga Journal website.

YOGA DIRECTORY

(Some of the listings in this directory came from the Yoga Journal resource directory online [www.yogajournal.com]. For more locations and contact information, please visit their site.)

ALABAMA
Yoga Connection, LLC
1067 Woodley Rd.
Montgomery, AL 36106
Phone: (334) 264-9642
www.yogamontgomery.com

ALASKA
The Yoga Studio (AK)
6921 Brayton Dr., Ste. 203
Anchorage, AK 99507
Phone: (907) 243-2846
yoginijt@aol.com

ARIZONA
The Yoga Experience
17 N. San Francisco St., Ste. 3C
Flagstaff, AZ 86001
Phone: (520) 774-9010

Yoga Oasis
2631 N. Campbell Ave.
Tucson, AZ 85701
Phone: (520) 322-6142
www.yogaoasis.com

ARKANSAS
Barefoot Studio
3604 Kavanaugh Blvd.
Little Rock, AR 72205
Phone: (501) 661-8005
www.barefootstudio.com

CALIFORNIA
Yoga in Motion
575 Lincoln St., Ste. 345
Napa, CA 94559
Phone: (707) 251-9642
www.yogainmotion.com

Moksha Yoga Shala
2940 Camino Diablo, Ste. 200
Walnut Creek, CA 94596
Phone: (925) 927-7279
www.horneryoga.com

Bikram's Yoga College of India
1862 South La Cienega
Los Angeles, CA 90035
Phone: (310) 854-5800

Maha Yoga
13050 San Vicente
Brentwood, CA 90049
Phone: (310) 899-0047

Self-Realization Fellowship
17190 Sunset Blvd.
Los Angeles, CA
Phone: (310) 454-4114

Open Door Yoga
1500 Castro St.
San Francisco, CA 94114
Phone: (415) 824-5657
www.opendooryoga.com

The Mindful Body
2876 California St.
San Francisco, CA 94115
Phone: (415) 931-2639
www.themindfulbody.com

Malibu Yoga
22333 Pacific Coast Hwy.
Malibu, CA
Phone: (310) 456-5772
www.malibuyoga.net

Free Spirit Studio
2629 Alta Arden
Sacramento, CA 95825
Phone: (916) 489-8780
www.freespiritstudio.com

Berkeley Yoga Center
1250 Addison St., Ste. 209
Berkeley, CA 94702
Phone: (510) 843-8784
www.berkeleyyoga.com

East West Yoga and Health Center
1356 Garnet Ave.
San Diego, CA 92109
Phone: (679) 687-7747
www.eastwestyoga.com

COLORADO

Iyengar Yoga Center of Denver
770 S. Broadway
Denver, CO 80209
Phone: (720) 570-9642
klaig@aol.com
www.iyengaryogacenter.com

Body Mind Dynamics
3055 Corona Trail, #304
Boulder, CO 80301
Phone: (303) 402-0443

The Aspen Yoga Studio
333 E. Durant Ave.
Aspen, CO 81612
Phone: (970) 920-0115
www.aspenyoga.net

CONNECTICUT

The Yoga Center of Greenwich
125 Greenwich Ave.
Greenwich, CT 06830
Phone: (203) 661-0092

Sun-to-Moon Yoga
2001 Whitney Ave.
New Haven, CT 06473
Phone: (203) 287-0216

YogaPuram
100 Allyn St., 3rd Fl.
Hartford, CT 06103
Phone: (860) 278-YOGA (9642)
www.yogapuram.com

D.C.

Ashtanga Yoga Center (D.C.)
4435 Wisconsin Ave. N.W.
Washington, DC 20016
Phone: (202) 342-6029
www.ashtangayogadc.com

The Dancing Heart Center for Yoga & The Art of Living
221 5th St. N.E.
Washington, DC 20002
Phone: (202) 544-0841
www.dancingheartyoga.com

DELAWARE

Wilmington Yoga
Wilmington, DE
Phone: (302) 777-3143
www.wilmingtonyoga.com

FLORIDA

Boca Yoga
450 N.E. 20th St.
Boca Raton, FL 33431
Phone: (561) 368-7368
bocayoga@yahoo.com

Medha Yoga & Healing Arts Inc.
915 N.E. 20th Ave.
Ft. Lauderdale, FL 33304
Phone: (954) 761-1989
www.medhayoga.com

Yoga Warehouse
508 S.W. Flagler Ave.
Ft. Lauderdale, FL 33301
Phone: (954) 525-7726
www.yogawarehouse.org

Yoga and Health Center of Orlando
14307 Tambourine Dr.
Orlando, FL 32837
www.edelyoga.com

Yoga Energy Center Inc.
624 1st Ave. S., Ste. 100
St. Petersburg, FL 33704
Phone: (727) 360-7870
www.yogaenergy.com

Synergy Yoga Center
435 Espanola Way
Miami Beach, FL 33139
Phone: (305) 538-7073
www.synergyyoga.org

GEORGIA

Atlanta Yoga
609 9th St. Northwest
Atlanta, GA 30318
Phone: (404) 892-7797

Java Devi Yoga Studio
312C North Highland Ave.
Atlanta, GA 30307
Phone: (404) 688-6757

Peachtree Yoga Center
6050 Andy Spring Circle
Atlanta, GA 30328
Phone: (404) 847-9642

HAWAII

Purple Yoga
P.O. Box 29645
Honolulu, HI 96820-2645
www.purpleyoga.com

Sweet Om Yoga
4-1495 Kuhio Hwy.
Kapaa, Kauai, HI 96746
Phone: (808) 823-9824
www.sweetomyoga.com

Maui Yoga Shala for the Body,
Mind and Soul
618 Hana Hwy.
Paia, Maui, HI 96779
www.maui-yoga.com

IDAHO
Boise Yoga Center
3113 Rose Hill
Boise, ID 83706
Phone: (208) 343-9786
www.boiseyogacenter.com

ILLINOIS
Moksha Yoga Center
700 N. Carpenter
Chicago, IL 60622
Phone: (312) 942-9642
www.mokshayoga.com

Priya Yoga Studio
One E. Oak St., Ste. 3W
Chicago, IL 60611
Phone: (312) 587-7492
www.priyayoga.com

N.U. Yoga Center
3047 N. Lincoln Ave., Ste. 320
Chicago, IL 60657
Phone: (773) 327-3650
www.yogamind.com

White Iris Yoga (IL)
1822 Ridge Ave.
Evanston, IL 60201
Phone: (847) 864-9987
www.whiteirisyoga.com

Namaste Yoga Center
2160 S. 6th St.
Springfield, IL 62703
Phone: (217) 698-8177
www.namasteyoga.com

INDIANA
The Yoga Studio (Indianapolis, IN)
2070 E. 54th St., Studio 12
Indianapolis, IN 46220
Phone: (317) 255-7363
sikesyoga@aol.com

IOWA
Serenity, Center for Yoga
5340 N. Park Pl. N.E.
Cedar Rapids, IA 52402
Phone: (319) 377-5300
www.serenity-inc.com

Anatoly's Spa
908 E. Market St.
Iowa City, IA 52245
Phone: (319) 354-3536
yogamovesme@aol.com

KANSAS
School of the Martial and
Meditative Arts
4009 S.W. 21st St.
Topeka, KS 66604
Phone: (785) 273-4343
prana_yama@yahoo.com

Barefoot Studio (KS)
8225 E. 35th St. N.
Wichita, KS 67235
Phone: (316) 636-YOGA (9642)
www.barefootstudio.net

KENTUCKY
The Yoga Center (KY)
432 E. Main St.
Bowling Green, KY 42101
Phone: (270) 746-9400

Yoga East, Inc. (E. Kentucky St.,
Louisville, KY)
1135 E. Kentucky St.
Louisville, KY 40204
Phone: (502) 585-9642
www.yogaeast.org

LOUISIANA
New Orleans Yoga Center
4842 Perrier St.
New Orleans, LA 70118
Phone: (504) 894-0024
www.neworleansyogacenter.com

MAINE
Portland Yoga Studio
616 Congress St.
Portland, ME 04103
Phone: (207) 797-5684
info@portlandyoga.com
www.portlandyoga.com

MARYLAND
Serenity Bay Yoga
3355 Arundel on the Bay Rd.
Annapolis, MD 21403
Phone: (410) 990-0909
www.serenitybayyoga.com

Yama Studio (yoga, ayurveda &
meditation arts)
2654 Maryland Ave.
Baltimore, MD 21218
Phone: (443) 662-YOGA
(9642)
www.yogasite.com/yama

MASSACHUSETTS
Dynamic Yoga
Cambridge, MA
Phone: (617) 983-8353
www.kurukulla.org

John Stasio and Associates
115 Newbury St., Ste. 204
Boston, MA 02116
Phone: (617) 522-5632
www.stasio.com

Bikram Yoga (MA)
108 Lincoln St., Loft 1A
Boston, MA 02111
Phone: (617) 556-9926
www.bikramyogaboston.com

The Yoga Studio (Boston, MA)
74 Joy St.
Boston, MA 02114
Phone: (617) 523-7138
www.yogastudio.org

The Yoga Studio & Namaste
Cafe
132 Adams St., Ste. 3
Newton, MA 02458
Phone: (617) 964-2985
www.yogawithjudi.com

Coolcat Yoga
Provincetown, MA 02657
Phone: (508) 487-7111
www.coolcatyoga.com

MICHIGAN
Yoga and Meditation
P.O. Box 2783
Ann Arbor, MI 48106
Phone: (734) 665-7801
www.yogaandmeditation.com

Isha Yoga Centre and Foundation
(MI)
Detroit, MI
Phone: (615) 665-3812
www.ishafoundation.org

Namaste Yoga, R.Y.T.
309 Troy St.
Royal Oak, MI 48067
Phone: (248) 399-9642
www.namaste-yoga.net

MINNESOTA
Minneapolis Yoga Workshop
810 W. 31st St.
Minneapolis, MN 55408
Phone: (612) 825-2554
www.mplsyogaworkshop.com

B.K.S. Iyengar Yoga Center
2736 Lyndale Ave. S.
Minneapolis, MN 55408
Phone: (612) 872-8708
chirh001@tc.umn.edu

St. Paul Yoga Center Inc.
1162 Selby Ave.
St. Paul, MN 55104
Phone: (651) 644-7141

MISSISSIPPI
Joyflow Yoga Center for Healing
558 Hwy. 51 N., Ste. D, Log
Village
Ridgeland, MS 39157
Phone: (601) 898-0300
www.joyflowyoga.com

MISSOURI
Heartland Yoga & Acupuncture
7216 Wornall Rd.
Kansas City, MO 64114
Phone: (816) 822-0500
coleton@solve.net

Yoga Gallery
2010 Baltimore, 4th Fl.
Kansas City, MO 64108
Phone: (816) 221-7323
hometown.aol.com/yogallery

Big Bend Yoga Center
88 N. Gore
St. Louis, MO 63119
Phone: (314) 918-YOGA
(9642)

MONTANA
Northern Lights Yoga
2751 Grizzly Gulch Dr.
Helena, MT 59601
Phone: (406) 449-2205
nly@qwest.net

Lotus Yoga
248A N. Higgins, #222
Missoula, MT 59802
Phone: (406) 721-1124
www.releasewithyoga.com

NEBRASKA
"Planet at Play"
1004 W. 9th St.
Grand Island, NE 68801
Phone: (308) 381-0254
www.planetatplay.com

NEVADA
The Hatha Yoga Center
7260 W. Lake Mead Blvd., Ste. 3
Las Vegas, NV 89128
Phone: (702) 233-9042

Active Yoga Studio
2605 S. Decatur Blvd., Ste. 214
Las Vegas, NV 89102
Phone: (702) 247-YOGA (9642)
activeyoga@aol.com

Mountain Spirit Yoga
Reno, NV
Phone: (775) 329-1999
1hume@sprynet.com

NEW HAMPSHIRE
Yoga & Meditation of Lebanon, NH
14 Green St.
Lebanon, NH 03766
Phone: (603) 448-1706
doreen.schweizer@valley.net

The Prana Studio for Yoga & Health
13 Sunnyside Dr.
Durham, NH 03824
Phone: (603) 868-6753

NEW JERSEY
First Street Yoga Studio
111 First St., #3-3A
Jersey City, NJ 07302
Phone: (201) 610-9737
www.firststreetyoga.com

SoHo Yoga
100 Valley Rd.
Montclair, NJ 07042
Phone: (973) 783-2269
www.sohoyoga.com

Princeton Center for Yoga & Health
Montgomery Commons
113 Commons Way
Princeton, NJ 08540
Phone: (609) 924-7294
www.princetonyoga.com

Dancing Foot Yoga
10 Broad St.
Red Bank, NJ 08750
Phone: (732) 219-6662
www.dancingfootyoga.com

Integrative Yoga Strategies
198 The Plaza
Teaneck, NJ 07666
Phone: (201) 833-8811
www.iysyoga.com

NEW MEXICO
YogaNow
215 Gold S.W.
Albuquerque, NM 87102
Phone: (505) 232-4717
www.yoganow.org

Yoga Source, Santa Fe
518 Old Sante Fe Trail
Santa Fe, NM 87501
Phone: (505) 982-0990
www.yogasource-santafe.com

Taos Yoga Center
4075 NDCBU
Taos, NM 87571
Phone: (505) 758-8007
www.sonyaluz.com

NEW YORK
The Body Shop
26 Newtown Ln.
East Hampton, NY 11937
Phone: (631) 324-6440

Yoga Shanti
75 Main St.
P.O. Box 2642
Sag Harbor, NY 11963
Phone: (631) 725-6424
www.yogashanti.com

Mind-Body Balance
759 President St.
Brooklyn, NY 11215
Phone: (718) 636-3950

Yoga Connection in Tribeca
145 Chambers St., 1st Fl.
New York, NY 10007
Phone: (212) 945-9642
www.yogaconnectionnyc.com

Integral Yoga Institute
227 W. 13th St.
New York, NY 10011
Phone: (212) 929-0586
www.integralyogaofnewyork.org

Laughing Lotus
55 Christopher St.
New York, NY 10014
Phone: (212) 414-2903
www.laughinglotus.com

Patanjali Yoga Shala
430 Broome St.
New York, NY 10012
Phone: (212) 431-3738

OM Yoga Center
135 W. 14th St., 2nd Fl.
New York, NY 10011
Phone: (212) 229-0267
www.omyoga.com

Sivananda Yoga Vedanta Center
234 W. 24th St.
New York, NY 10011

Bikram Yoga NYC
150 Spring St., 2nd Fl.
New York, NY 10012
Phone: (212) 245-2458
www.bikramyoganyc.com

Jivamukti Yoga Center
404 Lafayette St., 3rd Fl.
New York, NY 10003
Phone: (212) 295-6814
www.jivamuktiyoga.com

The Energy Center
53 Wyckoff St.
Brooklyn, NY 11201
Phone: (718) 243-1285
www.theenergycenter.com

East Meets West Yoga
220 Lexington Ave.
Buffalo, NY 14222
Phone: (716) 885-9100
www.eastmeetswestyoga.com

NORTH CAROLINA
The Yoga Loft (NC)
375 Depot St.
Asheville, NC 28804
Phone: (828) 254-8415
www.myyogaloft.com

Yoga Spot
501 Washington St., Ste. K
Durham, NC 27701
Phone: (919) 667-9642
www.yogaspot.com

Nirvana Yoga
Falls Village Shopping Ctr.
6677 Falls of the Neuse Rd., Ste. M
Raleigh, NC 27615
Phone: (919) 870-1754
www.nirvanayoga.com

OHIO
Earth & Sky Yoga
Cincinnati, OH
Phone: (513) 981-0113
www.earthandsky.ohgolly.com

Bhumi's Yoga and Wellness
Center
King James Plaza
25068 Center Ridge Rd.
Cleveland, OH 44145
Phone: (440) 899-9569
www.bhumiyoga.com

Yoga One
1780 W. Fifth Ave.
Columbus, OH 43212
Phone: (614) 487-YOGA (9642)
www.yogaone.org

OKLAHOMA
Yoga for Every Body (OK)
1416 E. 36th Pl.
Tulsa, OK 74105
Phone: (918) 748-YOGA (9642)

OREGON
The Sanctuary: A Center for
Yoga, Dharma & Healing Arts
4515 S.W. Corbett Ave.
Portland, OR 97201
Phone: (503) 552-YOGA (9642)
www.yogajoy.net

Julie Lawrence Yoga Center
1020 S.W. Taylor St., Ste. 780
Portland, OR 97205
Phone: (503) 227-5524
www.jlyc.com

Health & Fitness Yoga Center
510 S.W. 3rd Ave., Ste. 210
Portland, OR 97204
Phone: (503) 224-8611
www.holidaysyogacenter.com

The Movement Center: Yoga for
Everyone
1021 N.E. 33rd Ave.
Portland, OR 97232
Phone: (503) 231-0994
www.mcyoga.com

PENNSYLVANIA
New Hope Yoga Studio
104 Sunset Dr.
New Hope, PA 18938
Phone: (215) 862-6624
eleary@ptd.net

Moving Arts Studio of Mt. Airy
(Ma Ma)
6819 Greene St.
Philadelphia, PA 19119
Phone: (215) 842-1040

Yoga on Main
4363 Main St.
Philadelphia, PA 19127
Phone: (215) 482-7877
www.yogaonmain.com

Yoga Sadhana Studio
1113 E. Carson St.
Pittsburgh, PA 15203
Phone: (412) 481-YOGA (9642)
www.pittsburghyoga.com

The Movement Studio
2134 N. 2nd St.
Harrisburg, PA 17110
Phone: (717) 238-0357
www.themovementcenter.net

RHODE ISLAND
Anahata Yoga School
191 Nashua St.
Providence, RI 02904
Phone: (401) 274-5876
www.anahatayogaschool.com

The Yoga Studio & BodyMind
Therapies
84 Melrose St.
Providence, RI 02907
Phone: (401) 941-0032
www.bodymindri.com

SOUTH CAROLINA
Holy Cow Yoga & Holistic
Center
10 Windermere Blvd.
Charleston, SC 29407
Phone: (843) 769-2269
www.holycowyoga.com

SOUTH DAKOTA
Quantum Specialties
716 W. McClellan St.
Lead, SD 57754
Phone: (605) 722-3325
www.quantumspecialties.com

TENNESSEE
Eastern Sun Yoga Studio
3534 Forrest
Memphis, TN 38122
Phone: (901) 681-0009
www.easternsunyoga.com

Midtown Yoga
524 S. Cooper
Memphis, TN 38104
Phone: (901) 921-2517
www.midtownyoga.com

Yoga Source (TN)
209 10th Ave. S., Studio 126
Nashville, TN 37203
Phone: (615) 254-9642
www.yogasource-nashville.com

TEXAS
Blue Gecko Yoga
7801 Shoal Creek Blvd., #228
Austin, TX 78757-1029
Phone: (512) 452-6623
bluegeckoyoga@cs.com

YOGA YOGA
1700 S. Lamar
Austin, TX 78704
Phone: (512) 326-3900
www.yogayoga.net

Dallas Yoga Center
4525 Lemmon, Ste. 305
Dallas, TX 75219
Phone: (214) 443-9642
www.dallasyogacenter.com

Aum Yoga Studio
(formerly Center for Awareness)
2507 Lazydale Dr.
Dallas, TX 75228
Phone: (214) 324-9455
http://home.att.net/~aumyogastudio/page2.html

The Wellness Center
2481 Forest Park Blvd.
Ft. Worth, TX 76110
Phone: (817) 926-9642
www.yogadoctor.com

Yogapath
1454 FM 1960 W.
Houston, TX 77090
Phone: (281) 880-9443
www.theyogapath.com

Yoga Body—Houston
4040 Milam, Ste. 330
Houston, TX 77006
Phone: (713) 522-6080
www.yogabodyhouston.com

San Antonio Yoga
5225 McCullough Ave.
San Antonio, TX 78212
Phone: (210) 824-4225

UTAH
The Yoga Center (UT)
4689 S. Holladay Blvd.
Salt Lake City, UT 84117
Phone: (801) 277-9166
www.yogautah.com

Yoga Central
1550 E. 3300 S.
Salt Lake City, UT 84106
Phone: (801) 466-8324
www.yogacentral.com

VERMONT
Yoga Vermont
1 Mill St., Ste. A23
Burlington, VT 05401
Phone: (802) 660-9718
www.yogavermont.com

VIRGINIA
Sun & Moon Yoga Studio
2105 N. Pollard St.
Arlington, VA 22207
Phone: (703) 525-9642
www.sunandmoonstudio.com

Yoga Source (VA)
3122 W. Cary St., Ste. 220
Richmond, VA 23226
Phone: (804) 288-9642
www.yogarichmond.com

WASHINGTON
Seattle Holistic Center
7700 Aurora Ave. N.
Seattle, WA 98103
Phone: (206) 525-9035
holisticcenter@home.com
www.seattleholisticcenter.com

8 Limbs Yoga Center Inc.
500 E. Pike St.
Seattle, WA 98122
Phone: (206) 325-1511
www.eightlimbsyoga.com

Sadhana Yoga Studio
2218 3rd Ave. N.
Seattle, WA 98109
Phone: (206) 285-1491
www.sadhanayoga.com

Samadhi Yoga Center
1205 E. Pike St., #1B
Seattle, WA 98122
Phone: (206) 329-4070
www.samadhi-yoga.com

WISCONSIN
Bay Area Yoga Center
900 Cedar St.
Green Bay, WI 54301
Phone: (920) 435-1209
www.bayyoga.com

Well Within Collaborative
Wellness Center
4510 Regent St.
Madison, WI 53705
Phone: (608) 236-9138
www.wellwithinmadison.com

Stillpoint Yoga
7933 Stickney Ave.
Milwaukee, WI 53213
Phone: (414) 453-4407
stillpointyoga@hotmail.com

WYOMING
The Yoga Room (WY)
150 E. Hansen St.
Jackson, WY 83014
Phone: (307) 733-9260
snowdonyoga@earthlink.net

International
Future Yoga School
Casella Postale 36
Venice, Italy 30100
Phone: 011-39-041-277-0982
www.futureyoga.com

Downward Dog Yoga Centre
735 Queen St. West, 2nd Fl.
Toronto, M6J 1G1
Canada
Phone: (416) 703-8805
www.downwarddog.com

Bikram Yoga Montreal
721 Walker St.
Montreal, Quebec,
Canada
Phone: (514) 973-9642
www.bikramyogamtl.com

Chakrasana Yoga Studio
5122 Sherbrooke St. W., #102
Montreal, H4A 1T1
Canada
Phone: (514) 489-0862

Victoria Yoga Centre
Unit 592 #185-911 Yates St.
Victoria, V8V 4A8
Canada
Phone: (250) 386-YOGA (9642)
www.victoriayogacentre.com

**MOVEO Studio for Yoga,
Movement and Bodywork**
Tempelhofer Berg 7D
Berlin 10965
Germany
www.moveoberlin.de

Innergy Yoga Center
81 Hall East Row
Kensell Road, London W10
England
Phone: 011-44-20-8968-1178

Iyengar Yoga Vidyasthana
Centre de Yoga Iyengar de Paris
35 ave. Victor Hugo
Paris, 75116
France
Phone: 011-33-1-45-00-28-48

**International Yoga
Center/Ashtanga Yoga Shala
Tokyo**
Fukumura Ogikubo Bldg. 4P1
5-30-6 Ogikubo Suginami-ku
Tokyo, 167-0051
Japan
Phone: 011-81-3-5397-2741
kenergy99@hotmail.com

TriYoga (UK)
6 Erskine Rd., Primose Hill
London, NW3 3AJ
England
Phone: 011-44-207-483-3344
www.triyoga.co.uk

West London Yogashala
Basement 134 Gloucester Terr.
(entrance Cleveland Terr.),
Bayswater
London, W2 6HR
England
Phone: 011-44-20-7402-2217
yogashala@btinternet.com
Casa Shakti/Centro de Yoga

Calz. San Pedro 112 local 33
Monterrey, 64660
Mexico
Phone: 011-52-8335-9907
casashakti@yahoo.com

Institutions
Sivananda Yoga Vedanta Center
234 W. 24th St.
New York, NY 10011

The Ayurvedic Institute
P.O. Box 23455
Albuquerque, NM 87192
Phone: (505) 291-9698

The American Sanskrit Institute
73 Four Corners Rd.
Warwick, NY 10990

Ananda Ashram
Yoga Society of New York, Inc.
13 Sapphire Rd.
Monroe, NY 10950
Phone: (845) 782-5575

**Omega Institute for Holistic
Studies**
150 Lake Drive
Rhinebeck, NY 12572
Phone: (845) 266-4444
www.eomega.org

Brahmananda Ashram
Yoga Society of San Francisco, Inc.
2872 Folsom St.
San Francisco, CA 94110
Phone: (415) 285-5537

Kripalu Center for Yoga and Health
Box 793
Lenox, MA 01240
Phone: (800) 741-7353
www.kripalu.org

Iyengar Yoga Institute
27 W. 24th St., #800
New York, NY 10010
Phone: (212) 691-9642
www.yoga-ny.org

American Viniyoga Institute
P.O. Box 88
Makawao, HI 96768
Phone: (808) 572-1414
www.viniyoga.com

Siddha Yoga Foundation (SYDA Foundation)
P.O. Box 600
371 Brickman Road
South Fallsburg, NY 12747
Phone: (845) 434-2000
www.siddhayoga.org

Astanga Yoga Research Institute
Sri K. Pattabhi Jois
876/1 First Cross
Laxmipuram, 570004 Mysore
Karnataka, India
www.ayri.org

Krishnamacharya Yoga Mandiram
31 (Old #13) Fourth Cross Street
R K Nagar,
Chennai - 600 028, India
Phone: 91-44-4937998
www.kym.org

Websites
www.hindunet.org—a Hindu community and resource site on the net. This website provides many useful links and information from news to yellow pages to history and contemporary Hinduism.

www.vastuliving.com—Vastu consultant Kathleen Cox's site, dedicated to "Yoga for the Home"— creating a sacred space through the practice of Vastu.

www.americanbuddhistcenter.org— an online environment for the transmission, recognition, and promotion of Dharma, offering chants and online meditation practice.

www.yogajournal.com—the official website of the magazine *Yoga Journal*.

www.self-realization.com/yoga directory.htm—one of many online yoga directories with national and international listings for yoga studios, accessible according to type and region.

www.tibethouse.org—the site of the New York–based Tibet House, a Tibetan institution dedicated to presenting and preserving Tibetan civilization, culture, and wisdom.

BIBLIOGRAPHY

Batchelor, Martine. *Meditation for Life*. Boston, Wisdom Publications, 2001.

Beversluis, Joel, ed. *Sourcebook of the World's Religions: An Interfaith Guide to Religion and Spirituality*. California, New World Library, 2000.

Bouldrey, Brian, ed. *Traveling Souls: Contemporary Pilgrimage Stories*. San Francisco, Whereabouts Press, 1999.

Chödrön, Pema. *Start Where You Are: A Guide to Compassionate Living*. Boston, Shambhala, 1994.

Cope, Stephen. *Yoga and the Quest for the True Self*. New York, Bantam Books, 1999.

Cox, Kathleen. *Vastu Living*. New York, Marlowe & Company, 2000.

de Bary, William Theodore, ed. *The Buddhist Tradition in India, China and Japan*. New York, Vintage Books, 1972.

Déchanet, J.-M., O.S.B. *Christian Yoga*. New York, Harper and Brothers Publishers, 1960.

Desikachar, T. K. V. *Health, Healing, and Beyond: Yoga and the Living Tradition of Krishnamacharya*. New York, Aperture, 1998.

————. *The Heart of Yoga: Developing a Personal Practice*. Vermont, Inner Traditions International, 1999.

Dikshit, Sudhakar S., ed. *I Am That: Talks with Nisargadatta Maharaj*. Durham, North Carolina, Acorn Press, 1973.

Embree, Ainslie T., ed. *The Hindu Tradition: Readings in Oriental Thought*. New York, Vintage Books, 1972.

Feuerstein, Georg, Ph.D. *The Yoga Tradition: Its History, Literature, Philosophy and Practice*. Prescott, Arizona, Hohm Press, 1998.

Flood, Gavin. *An Introduction to Hinduism*. Cambridge, England, Cambridge University Press, 1996.

Fontana, David. *The Secret Language of Symbols: A Visual Key to Symbols and Their Meanings*. San Francisco, Chronicle Books, 1994.

Fraser, Tara. *Total Yoga: A Step-by-Step Guide to Yoga at Home for Everybody*. London, Thorsons, 2001.

Hanh, Thich Nhat. *Living Buddha, Living Christ*. New York, Riverhead Books, 1995.

————. *The Miracle of Mindfulness: An Introduction to the Practice of Meditation*. Boston, Beacon Press, 1975.

Hope, Jane. *The Secret Language of the Soul: A Visual Guide to the Spiritual World*. San Francisco, Chronicle Books, 1997.

Hope-Murray, Angela, and Tony Pickup. *Discover Ayurveda*. Berkeley, Ulysses Press, 1998.

Hopkins, Thomas J. *The Hindu Religious Tradition*. California, Belmont, 1971.

Iyengar, B. K. S. *Light on Yoga*. New York, Schocken Books, 1979, revised edition.

Iyengar, Geeta S. *Yoga: A Gem for Women*. Spokane, Washington, Timeless Books, 1990.

Johnson, Will. *The Posture of Meditation: A Practical*